BREAKING CONVENTION:
PSYCHEDELIC PHARMACOLOGY
FOR THE 21ST CENTURY

Lead Editor: Ben Sessa
Co-Editors: David Luke, Cameron Adams, David King, Aimee Tollan, Nikki Wyrd

A CIP catalogue record for this book is available from the British Library.

ISBN: 978-1-907222-55-9

Distributed by The MIT Press, Cambridge, Massachusetts. And London, England.
Printed and bound in Great Britain by TJ International Ltd. Padstow.

Strange Attractor Press
BM SAP, London, WC1N 3XX, UK
www.strangeattractor.co.uk

BREAKING CONVENTION: PSYCHEDELIC PHARMACOLOGY FOR THE 21ST CENTURY

LEAD EDITOR: BEN SESSA

CO-EDITORS: DAVID LUKE, CAMERON ADAMS, DAVID KING, AIMEE TOLLAN, NIKKI WYRD

BREAKING CONVENTION: PSYCHEDELIC PHARMACOLOGY FOR THE 21ST CENTURY

INTRODUCTION:
RE-BRANDING PSYCHEDELICS—
ONE HAIRCUT AT A TIME

It is a great pleasure to introduce *Breaking Convention: Psychedelic Pharmacology for the 21st Century,* the third instalment of Breaking Convention essays. Proceedings come from twenty-five of the superb speakers at our summer meeting in Greenwich, London in 2015. And what an event it was! Another wonderful rag-tag army of divergent disciplines, sliding over one another in a primordial soup of creative lysergic academia. From suited scientists to bare-torsoed hippies, everyone welcome, every viewpoint valid and all ideas up for discussion. Or are they? In this (potentially unpopular) introductory essay I will reflect upon this issue of schism; the differences between opinion, beliefs, facts and realities. It is, I believe, of utmost importance that we find a common voice and move as a cohesive group towards a non-prohibition world.

We all have our opinions; we all have principles. Try as we might to be cohesive, with such a varied range of positions, how are we to find an answer to that elusive question: What is Psychedelic? Perhaps none of us has the slightest clue how to best describe the experience itself? Indeed, it is fair to ask why we should bother anyway? But we could —*should*—in my opinion (there's that word again!) attempt a uniting acceptance that whatever is going on, it is a pretty good thing and we would like to see more of it; without being prosecuted. After fifteen years in psychedelic research as a medical doctor I am increasingly confused. And I think it all comes down to haircuts. Let me explain.

It can be difficult keeping up the appearance of a respectable medical doctor whilst also pursuing psychedelic research. Sitting in hospital board meetings or in front of ethics committees trying to convince one's conservative clinical colleagues about the healing potential of psychedelic drugs is a challenge. Many of my colleagues think I am mad. The propaganda success of the War on Drugs has poisoned the minds of many intelligent thinkers. Drugs are bad > Psychedelics are drugs > Psychedelics are bad. Warning me of 'career suicide', they suggest instead I prostitute myself to the Big Pharma pimps and research something more wholesome and proper, like antidepressants. They look at the tie-dye and dreadlocked hair of the psychedelic community and laugh. The Industry has nothing to fear from that lot. These hippies have spent fifty years campaigning on cognitive liberty and their 'right to get high' and it has got them precisely... nowhere. Almost all psychedelics, almost everywhere in the world, remain banned. And a good thing too.

So, as a concurrent member of the psychedelic community, I turn to them for support. Come the weekend, I am fraternising at raves and festivals, jabbering wildly around campfires at dawn with other saucer-eyed nutcases. And then it is *them* trying to convince me that it is *they* that have the answers; and those pesky doctors and scientists should stay out of the debate. I meet one well-meaning psychonaut after another, frustrating me with their pseudoscientific half-knowledge of chemistry and pharmacology gleaned from YouTube. I get dragged into debates about the 'medical model', told I am a pawn of the system and am simply toeing the government line with my medical practice. 'Thing is, man, *we know* the answers... we don't need your science, man. LSD is the answer. You just have to ask her.'

What, then, to do? Fence sitting is not an option. It leads to painful buttock problems. Rather, finding a way to straddle the complexities of contemporary science and the swirling world of culture, art, religion, society and politics is required. A mighty task. It's enough to turn one to drugs. However, for me, it is exactly this challenging opportunity, immersed in a field of study encompassing so many contrasts and controversies, that makes it so exciting. Criticism of the medical model is essential. Scientists have been the guardians of objective reality for too long. Science-driven consumerist technology creates separation from our souls and from one another. Despite the promised interconnectivity of the internet, we are at risk of producing a generation of people who now sit in trains, airports and even their family homes, detached from one another, staring silently into screens, each of us alone, obese, bored, apathetic and spiritually vacuous. Pretending we are winners because we can collectively 'like' someone else's equally half-understood oversimplification of complex issues. Meanwhile, less than three clicks of a mouse away, a growing generation of starving children are blown apart by wars, drowning in social inequality on a scale never imagined. The losers of this great social experiment. So, come on, psychonauts, tell me, *how* is LSD going to solve this problem?

What we have here, folks, is a lack of organisation, communication and dissemination of psychedelic information. Psychedelic science has proved beyond doubt that these compounds are overwhelmingly safe, and should be employed throughout clinical medicine right now, without delay. They work. They provide a much-needed breakthrough for those thousands of people suffering refractory mental disorders. We know this. So why are health authorities not queuing up to open ayahuasca clinics, ibogaine retreats, MDMA gyms and LSD spas? I would propose that the answer to that question—and responsibility for why psychedelics have remained marginalised and unnecessarily outlawed for so long—lies with you, psychonauts. You blew it, man. You've had two generations to find a clever way to translate the psychedelic experience into something transformative to save humanity from destruction and what have you got to show for it? Psytrance? It is seventy years since Albert's bike ride and less than 2% of the UK population have ever tried that predominantly harmless, potentially beneficial, substance: LSD. I would not call that a successful outcome for dissemination of good news.

It is time to up our game and, in my opinion, pin our flags more firmly to the mast of science. Arguably, scientists have done more in the last ten years to open the mainstream debate about the safety and benefit of psychedelics than any of the socio-culturally mediated dissemination attempts of the previous decades. It was science that got medicinal cannabis into American states. Science has launched projects with LSD, psilocybin, DMT and MDMA all over the world. For the first time ever, we are getting positive media coverage describing safe psychedelic drug use in a legal setting. And, if anything can, it will be science that pulls down the pillars of prohibition.

But science is dull. At its heart is a boring methodical process; one that requires repetition, time and effort. Science lacks class and style, colour and romance. But it gives us data. And when it comes to politicians making decisions about important social issues, data is the best weapon we have to change hearts and minds.

Or... is it? Because here we meet another problem. Although, as stated, we have established the efficacy and safety of psychedelics, we still seem to be hitting a brick wall. Politicians are not listening. As a scientist interested in drug development this is incredibly frustrating. Over the years many other drugs have found their way to becoming prescription medicines on the back of far flimsier studies than those to which we have subjected MDMA, LSD, psilocybin and cannabis in recent years. Therefore, it appears data alone is not enough, as Professor David Nutt discovered in 2010. He provided the British government with a plethora of meticulous, peer-reviewed data about the safety and efficacy of MDMA, requesting a change in its scheduling and permission to get lifesaving research underway. What did the government do? They sacked him. And that fiasco leaves me, as a scientist, feeling somewhat impotent. What am I to do in my own humble practice if a luminary like Nutt can be so cynically swept aside? How can I make progress in this field? Data and science are all I have. I don't know how to battle with forces of authority who don't play by the rules of science.

Oh, dear. Now what are we going to do?! Neither the hippies and their campfire cognitive liberty calls, nor the sober and rigorous

Nutt, playing by the rules with his scientific evidence, have worked. This means we need an entirely new approach; something creative that spans science and culture. What psychedelics need, I propose, as a matter of utter urgency, is a facelift. Forget data and forget our cognitive rights. What we need now is simply *good PR*. Not necessarily Saatchi and Saatchi (although that might be interesting), but rather the skill and ingenuity of the media-savvy. People who can massage the masses. And for this reason, I am thrilled by the work of Breaking Convention, the Psychedelic Society, the Psychedelic Press, MAPS, Heffter, Beckley and all the other outlets appearing around the world working towards effecting real change. These are not fringe groups living on small-holdings in Wales, shunning society in their pursuit of personal psychedelic salvation. Rather, we are out shouting in the cities, making noise, getting things done and refusing to go away. It's time to end the apathy of wasted decades doused in patchouli oil. Goodbye 1970s psychedelia. It's time to break windows. (Pacifistically, of course).

I do not believe that bringing psychedelics into mainstream consciousness is a sell-out. Sometimes underground therapists criticise the likes of MAPS, Heffter and the Beckley-Imperial research programs. 'We already have MDMA, man,' they tell me. 'We don't need your studies. Come to my place in California and I can treat you. The underground scene is alive and kicking.' OK, fine. That is all very well for those fortunate few people with the necessary knowledge and financial resources. But there are some 60,000 cases of untreated PTSD in the UK. They can't all fly off to California or spend four months in the Peruvian jungle to get their medicine. I see an unhelpful undercurrent of arrogant exclusivity that exists within some parts of today's psychedelic community. A serious barrier to many people who could benefit from these medicines. The community imagines itself as 'right on' and open, but it, just like clinical medicine, is also rife with rigid stereotypes that exclude access to many. Chakras, energy levels, crop circles, UFOs, entities, incense, tie-dye, long hair, fractals, crystals, indigo children and perinatal matrices are not everybody's cup of mushroom tea. When

I look at the patients in my clinics what I see are ordinary, mostly poor and uneducated, everyday people. They have shaved heads and tattoos, wear tracksuits, listen to Capital Radio, smoke fags, drink beer, watch *X-Factor* and eat junk food. Mandalas and sitar music are not their world. Yet it is precisely these people, my worthy patients whom I respect so deeply, that are most in need of these magic medicines.

So, to the book you are holding. Here we deliver the message to dissolve these barriers:

- **Sam Gandy**'s essay, *Who's Tripping Whom?*, reflects on humanity's potential to destroy itself and half of the planet's species and asks whether the symbiotic role played by psychedelic plants and fungi might teach us how to survive.
- **Allan Badiner** continues this theme in *Psychedelics in the Anthropocene*, exploring the system of ethics apparent in both Buddhist and psychedelic experience. Can psychedelics offer the rapid mental evolution and social change required?
- **Friederike Fischer**'s essay, *Risks and Harms on Psychedelics*, wisely reminds us not to disregard the wealth of experience of underground therapists.
- **Tharcila Chaves**, in *Special Features of Special K*, gives us the pharmacology of ketamine and a review of recent clinical studies.
- **John Constable** and his *Acid Mediumship: Goose and Crow* leaps into the abyss with a poetic description of a heroic dose of LSD, via verse and visions, in praise of the ancient outcast spirit.
- **Lorna Olivia O'Dowd** in *Self, Meaning and Transformation*, describes a journey of family trauma, mental health problems, separation and loss that carries her subject to the door of ayahuasca.
- **Rick Doblin**, the CEO of MAPS, is *Becoming Conventional*, as the golden goal of MDMA licensing looms ever closer; reassuring us the medicine will be outside of corporate pharma and accessible to all.

- **Amanda Feilding,** whilst heralding the successes of recent developments in research and policy reforms, reminds us in *Research at the Frontiers of Prohibition* that there is still much work to be done.
- **Mike Crowley,** with mushroom spectacles in place, in *Psychedelic Mushrooms: An Ancient Women's Secret?* finds ancient Goddess pharmacologists at every twist and turn.
- **Robert Dickins,** the brains behind the Psychedelic Press, with *In a Song of Insurrection and Madness,* traces how acidic poetry has conquered the barrier of ineffability.
- **Luke Goaman-Dodson,** with *The Real Secret of Magic,* describes a Burroughs-McKenna deconstructed interzone of hyper-reality cut-ups inhabited by octopi and Scientologists.
- **Ido Hartogsohn** takes us back to the 1950s with *A Psychedelic Technology,* insightfully reflecting that psychedelics are indeed a slippery fish, creating inevitable pitfalls for objective categorisation.
- **Scott Hill** provides perspective with *Archetypes and the Collective Unconscious,* revealing the psychedelic community's peculiar embrace of Jung, despite the psychoanalyst's own apparent distaste for the drugs themselves.
- **Will Rowlandson,** in *Altered States of Unconscious,* inserts the elves and entities that no self-respecting book on psychedelics dare leave out, and questions their meaning and relevance in relation to the DMT experience.
- **David E. Nichols,** renowned chemist who cut his teeth with Shulgin in the 1970s, churns out new molecules in *Random Selections: From Research Tools to Research Chemicals.*
- **Jennifer Lyke and Julia Kuti** describe a *Case Report of a High Frequency, Non-Clinical Hallucinogen User,* who took the unusual decision to consume high dose psilocybin daily for ten months and in the process jumped, unscathed, free from the hamster wheel of life.
- **Michael Montagne,** in *Saving and Archiving the World Literature on Psychedelic Drugs,* stresses the importance of collecting and archiving

the history of psychedelic experiences and literature using Google's Ngram Viewer—an essential task, leaving no left turn unstoned.

- **Jonathan Newman** wonders what a freed-weed future might be like in *Transgression and Economy During Drug Reform,* providing models and options from free-markets to corporate interventions. Coming soon to a supermarket shelf near you.
- **Carl Ruck**, in *Restoring Ancient Mysteries,* uncovers the secrets of Eleusis with his exploration of wild grasses and fungal corn kernels at the table of Demeter and Dionysus.
- **Dale Pendell** and his *Lunar Meanders* provides confusion and contusion about collusion with the delusion, which is exactly what we need.
- **Alan Piper**, in *Psychedelics, Transgression and the End of History,* explores the forbidden nature of psychedelics and ponders whether becoming mainstream risks losing their mojo.
- **Graham St John**, with *Pineal Enigma,* gives us a Strassmanian journey on the back of the spirit molecule to investigate endogenous psychedelic beliefs.
- **Bruce Rimmel** tackles more big questions in *On Vision and Being Human.* What is art? What is reality? And whatever the 'otherness' is, to limit ourselves from dwelling there could be folly in the extreme.
- **Iker Puente** reminds us it is not all about drugs. In *Subjective Effects of Holotropic Breathwork,* he compares Griffiths' psilocybin participants with a group undergoing Breathwork and reveals surprising results when it comes to mystical experiences.
- **Tim Read**, in *Psychedelics and Numinous Experience,* takes us on Hofmann's bicycle into Plato's cave, where he encounters shadows and rebirth and ends up with angels amongst the stars.

Yes, *Breaking Convention: Psychedelic Pharmacology for the 21st Century* is full of divergent views and opinions. As we progress towards the quantum there are no more truths in science than there are in any other field of study. We find equal measures of ignorance and arrogance on both sides of the debate. Enthusiastic but non-trained pseudo-experts peddling half-truths about complex subjects are no better than the readily maligned short-sighted doctors and scientists who cannot see beyond the end of their stethoscopes. Rather than be overly accepting of such erroneous views and say 'both are valid,' in my opinion we should be stricter and more accurately describe both positions as invalid. Neither should be accepted.

Does this mean there a schism imminently emerging in the field of psychedelics? Are we about to see breakaway factions battling it out at psychedelic conferences for their place on the astral plane? Turf wars over $5-HT_{2A}$ agonist trading rights? Are we looking at a future where the men in suits, with their talks of receptors and fMRIs, will no longer share the platform with Salvia Spirits and the fields of morphic resonance? I seriously hope not.

After all, this situation is not new. The *Are You Experienced?* approach has been there since the beginning. The moment Hofmann stumbled back into the lab after his bicycle experience, and he and Stoll sat down with the others at Sandoz to discuss who in the department was going to try this new LSD-25 next and, crucially, who was *not*, the schism was in place. The rapid growth of ayahuasca interest in recent years has created a new version of this phenomenon. Is your Aya experience better because you spent four months squatting in a Peruvian jungle whereas I had mine in a kitchen in Swindon with products bought online? Quite possibly, at some levels, but not to the extent that my experience has no validity whatsoever. Exclusivity amongst the psychedelic community needs to be tackled. It is snobbishness in the extreme to say otherwise; and such attitudes risk undermining accessibility to psychedelics for everyone. Let us not give our critics any extra excuses to rubbish our subject.

Psychedelics rely on cohesion for future generations. They have always had an ability to drive wedges between young and old. Leary said not to trust anyone over 45. (He was, of course, in his late forties at the time—always the joker). But he was rightly highlighting the apparently natural trajectory towards conservativism that comes with increasing age. The pseudo-psychedelic children of the 1960s became the yuppies of the 1980s; the greatest prohibitionists of the last 1,000 years. We must not let that happen to us in the 2050s—I don't think humanity could take it again.

Psychedelics need normalisation. Neither venerated as solely mystical and spiritual, only to be used in exclusive circumstances by exclusive intellectuals (as Huxley proposed); but neither should they be prohibited and maligned. They should simply be used; in whatever way people feel is right for them. This normalisation, outing approach, is essential. Let's look at what we can learn from other slandered minority groups. Although the loud exchanges, marches in the streets and placard waving of the 1960s and '70s were an essential part of various minority groups' liberation, it was not until diversity became normal and, dare I say it, appropriately boring and ordinary, in the 1990s, that we started seeing barriers coming down and a move towards equality. Of course, homophobia, sexism and racism are far from eradicated; tackling discrimination is a work in progress. Diversity matters, and psychedelic history, like most history, which is written by the likes of Lewin, Hofmann, Heffter, Huxley, Leary, Whitehead, Bergson, James, Havelock Ellis and the rest, is sadly primarily represented by middle class old white men. This *must* change. This includes daring to criticise those indigenous cultures—whilst acknowledging the skilful means by which they have integrated psychedelic use within their social systems —where sexism, racism and homophobia are often abundant. To deny this is to fall into the patronising trap of the noble savage and devalue what must be a global jump forward into the future—not a pathetic fall backwards into a far from perfect past.

Given such a poor outcome after seventy years of attempted psychedelicization of this destructive post-modern world, there cannot be many objections to considering a process of rebranding. Brave steps and left-field suggestions are welcomed. Everything is up for grabs and anything is possible. Perhaps the concept of 'MAPS Corp' is not as sinister as it sounds when one reads what is being proposed. Accessibility and dissolution of boundaries are the goals. Freedom from prosecution and the provision of small, non-profit independently run global cottage industries for psychedelic users is not, in my opinion, a bad direction to imagine. So, let's be shrewd as we go forward. The truth is that tie-dye and dreads will not get you through the door at Number 10 to even begin the conversation about psychedelic liberation with those in political power. A suit and neat haircut might. True, once in, we will still be met with stigmatising barriers of fear and misinformation, but at least we will have a (non-sandaled) foot in the door.

I conclude, however, with the admission that I say all this, of course, because I am a bald man who'd happily give up all this medicine malarkey tomorrow for a full head of dreads. In the meantime, psychonauts, just in case you are right and I am wrong, let's continue to ask LSD.

Enjoy the book!

WHO'S TRIPPING WHOM?

SAM GANDY

Man has had a profound impact on the ecology of the planet since our rise to dominance, becoming masters of shaping the world around us and bending nature to our whims. Many plants and fungi have grown strong associations with our species. Although unable to move, plants have managed to exploit animals into pollinating them and spreading their genes far and wide. Animals are exploited in the movement of plant seeds and fungal spores, so as to spread their influence further. When Man enters this picture, things become yet more complex. Through our long-term association with plants and fungi, we have discovered a vast array of species we consider valuable for a multitude of different reasons; as foods, building materials, medicines, poisons and intoxicants. Any species we deem to be of value have tended to benefit in their association with us, by our spreading them far beyond what their natural range would otherwise have been, and often by our manipulation of the surrounding ecology to provide them with optimal habitat while markedly reducing their competition with species we find less favourable. Due to our profound and far reaching modification of global ecology, we are now entering the Anthropocene, the age of Man, and this is coinciding with the sixth great mass extinction of life on this planet. Never before in the planet's history has a single species wielded such an awesome and terrible power over all life.

Plants and fungi comprise very ancient forms of life that lack the ability to flee predators so over evolutionary time they have become master chemical alchemists so as to defend themselves. Due to the evolutionary interconnectedness of all life, a number of plant defensive compounds share a close resemblance to, or may be identical to, endogenous human neurochemistry. A number of plants produce DMT, 5-MeO-DMT and bufotenine, all of them comprising some of the most powerful psychedelic substances known, and all of them known to be trace endogenous components of human neurochemistry. The psilocybin found in species of a certain genus of fungi bears a very close resemblance to both DMT and serotonin, an evolutionarily ancient neurotransmitter that plays a key role in brain and nervous system function in humans. The endogenous MAOI compound pinoline bears a close resemblance to harmaline and the beta-carboline alkaloids found in the ayahuasca (*Banisteriopsis caapi*) vine and Syrian rue (*Peganum harmala*). In effect, these plants and fungi have developed means to hack animal nervous systems.

Fungi are considered very simple organisms, and yet are fully capable of taking over much more complex organisms and bending them to their whims. One such example are *Cordyceps* species, which are parasitic fungi that feed on insects. When *Cordyceps* infects ants, the fungus wrests control of their nervous systems, forcing them to climb high up in vegetation, before then clamping down with their jaws to a branch. If another ant encounters an infected ant acting strange, it will immediately grab it and remove it from the vicinity of the colony and dump it on the ground. The *Cordyceps* forces the ant to climb high and then lock down securely so the spores produced by the fruiting body that emerges from the ant's head have the maximum potential area of distribution, so as to infect as many new ant hosts as possible.

Psychedelics, on their most superficial but nevertheless universal level, have a tendency to increase people's aesthetic appreciation for nature, and on a deeper level, put us in touch with nature in a profound way, with many people reporting a deep felt sense of oneness, unity and interconnectedness with the natural world. Such experiences can and do reinforce people's ecological awareness and concern for the natural world, as discussed by Krippner et al.,[1] and such insights are also linked to other human transcendent experiences, such as the near death experience. Human experimentation with psychedelics, at least in the Western world, exploded in the 1960s, and this coincides with the time that the spores of the ecological movement germinated and set forth their mycelial tendrils as explored by Doblin et al.,[2] while the hippie counterculture was embarking on the back-to-the-land movement, as mentioned by Rome.[3]

Research by Lerner et al.[4] and Studerus et al.[5] has shown that the self-reported beliefs and values of psychedelic users indicate a higher environmental concern than non-drug users or users of other substances, although it remains unclear whether this concern preceded the psychedelic experience or resulted from it, as observed by Maclean et al.[6] The late, great Dr Albert Hofmann perceived his creation LSD as making one aware of 'the magnificence of nature and of the animal and plant kingdom' and humanity's role in relation to nature.[7]

LSD has certainly had a widely felt impact on people's ecological perceptions. Former Merry Prankster Stewart Brand had the insight during an LSD trip in 1966 that humans had been to space, and yet no one had thought of taking a photograph of the Earth from space yet. Following this insight, he campaigned to make this happen, printing badges with the question "We've gone to space—Why do we have no photos of the whole Earth from space?" on them, sending them to Congress, and two years later in 1968 the Apollo 8 astronauts took arguably one of the most profound photographs ever taken, of the earthrise from the moon's surface. This stunning photograph was also a symbol and testament to how far we had come as a species, and became a powerful symbol of the ecological movement, and a year after this photo was taken, World Peace Day was founded.

Some of the founders of the Biosphere 2 project—the largest and most ambitious ecological experiment and semi self-sustaining ecosystem in the world—considered psychedelics as key inspirations. John P. Allen had a peyote vision in a Huichol Indian ceremony that was a pivotal experience for him, and engineer Mark Van Thillo wanted to try and bridge ecology with technology, seeing them as one and the same, via his use of psychedelics.

LSD also had a profound effect on the concept of deep ecology. Philosophers Arne Naess & John Seed considered their experience with LSD as highly influential on their thinking, as discussed by Schroll et al.[8] The concept of deep ecology concerns the appreciation of life in all its forms, that life has an inherent value beyond human needs, and living in equilibrium with that in mind should be a priority in life. Such a view is clearly in stark contrast to that held by the Abrahamic religious view of nature being something separate from us, of Man being something distinct and elevated beyond it and nature being there solely to be exploited how we see fit. This view, which regrettably still appears to hold sway in much of the world, may be a core reason behind the disconnection between Man and Nature, and all the damage to both that results from it.

Of all the plants that have benefited through an association with Man, none have gained more and played such a pivotal role in the rise of human civilisation than the grasses. Domestication of grasses such as rice, wheat, oats and maize lies at the foundation of human civilisation around the world. These plants, in effect, domesticated us by causing us to largely reject a nomadic hunter-gatherer existence in favour of a more sedentary, agricultural based life. For the first time in human history, people began to live together in larger and larger groups than they ever could before. By having a dependable food source on our doorstep, as a species we suddenly had more time on our hands, a division of labour resulted, and human culture and religion followed in its wake. We have chopped down forests and altered our surrounding ecology to an incredible degree to provide habitat for our favoured grasses at the expense of many other species that share the biosphere. These grasses included the species grown for food, as well as grass pastures which sustain our livestock. From these grassy habitats have emerged some powerful and important psychedelic fungi.

The liberty cap (*Psilocybe semilanceata*) is a species that is widespread in temperate parts of the world. It is one of the more common and most potent of psilocybin mushrooms known. The fungus is saprobic, the mycelium feeding on decaying grass roots. The grass habitat within which this species thrives has done very well due to human influence, and open grassland is a great deal more common than it otherwise would be. Furthermore, the species thrives in nitrogen rich pastureland fertilised with dung, although it is not directly associated with dung. Thus our manipulation of our ecology in this manner has vastly increased suitable habitat for this species, while at the same time increasing the likelihood of human encounters with it. *Psilocybe mexicana,* an important and widely used species in central America, cherished by the Aztecs and the Mazatec, also appears to favour human made habitats, such as along trails and roads, and in meadows and cornfields, and in grassy areas bordering deciduous woodland. The species *Psilocybe cubensis* has spread so widely around the world in tropical and subtropical regions that it isn't entirely clear where its original native range is. Due to its coprophilic or dung loving nature it has done very well following our domestication of a number of bovine species, and is widespread in subtropical and tropical pastures all over the world. The coprophilic and highly potent *Panaeolus* fungus genus has also benefitted through our actions.

Some grasses themselves are known to be potent psychedelics. *Phalaris* is a widespread group of grasses and some species such as *P. aquatica, P. brachystachys* and *P. arundinacea* have been found to contain high levels of tryptamine psychedelics such as DMT and 5-MeO-DMT. They have found use in ayahuasca analogue concoctions by intrepid psychonauts in recent times. *Phalaris* species such as *P. aquatica* and *P. arundinacea* have also been found to be highly invasive species in some parts of the world, thriving in disturbed areas, and members of this group have certainly benefitted through Man's actions on the biosphere.

LSD is a semi synthetic derivative of alkaloids from the fungus ergot (*Claviceps purpurea*). Like *P. semilanceata, C. purpurea* is another species that lives in close association with grasses and has done very well via our actions on the environment. The grasses in question are this time arable instead of pastoral, with the fungus being a parasite on the ears of cereals such as rye and related plants. Man has known of ergot for some time, and cases of ergot poisonings were not uncommon in the Middle Ages. It is unlikely that the invention and discovery of the very powerful psychedelic compound LSD would have occurred were it not for our domestication of grasses and manipulation of our surrounding ecology.

Salvia divinorum is considered an atypical psychedelic (which in scientific terms means something that is very, very strange). The Mexican Mazatec Indians who use it claim it is not from there and that it comes from elsewhere. It is rare in the wild, inhabiting a few ravines in central Mexico. Its biological origin remains somewhat a mystery. It is possibly a cultigen, and produces very few fertile seeds and reproduces via cloning; growing and then falling over and producing new plant growth from the old. As a species it has certainly benefited through an association with Man, often being planted around Mazatec dwellings, and it seems to thrive in captivity.

Visionary fungi have benefitted markedly through our association with trees. The fly agaric *Amanita muscaria* lives in symbiotic mycorrhizal association with pine trees, and through our actions with forestry has spread to many parts of the world unintentionally, and should be considered a cosmopolitan species, as mentioned by Geml et al.[9] The wood loving Psilocybes such as *P. cyanescens* and *P. azurescens* are among the most potent psilocybin-containing mushrooms known and have also benefitted markedly through our actions manipulating our surrounding ecology. These species would have occupied highly specialised niches previously, but due to actions of forestry and the ability of their spores to travel far and wide, they have benefited vastly via spreading through wood chips. Thus, on a global scale, our species' modification of our surrounding ecosystems can be seen as increasing both habitat and the likelihood of encounters with these psychedelic fungi. It is interesting to note the ability of these species to reliably enhance aesthetic appreciation of nature and ecological awareness in the humans that consume them, while having a tendency to proliferate in ecologically disturbed areas. Furthermore, the cultivation of Psilocybes around the world and deliberate seeding of wood chips with psilocybe mycelium has only assisted in their spread. Mycologist Paul

Stamets has referred to the wood loving psilocybes as anthropophilic in nature, but this description applies to all the species discussed here to some degree. So what may have evolved as some kind of defensive compound inferring evolutionary advantages on the fungal species in question seems to have further evolutionary benefits once Man enters the picture.

Other visionary plants have benefitted from us in a global sense. Syrian rue (*P. harmala*), cannabis (*Cannabis spp.*) and tobacco (*Nicotiana spp.*) are all ruderal plants, thriving on disturbed ground and areas associated with human activity. The Rastafari movement has long considered cannabis a sacrament that brings them 'closer to the earth' as discussed by Lee.[10] The psychedelic ergoline alkaloid contacting plants, the Morning Glory (*Ipomoea purpurea*) and the Hawaiian Baby Woodrose (*Argyreia nervosa*), have profoundly benefited through the actions of Man, the former species being naturalised throughout warm temperate and subtropical parts of the world, having spread well beyond its native Mexico and Central America. *A. nervosa* has been introduced to Hawaii, Africa and the Caribbean and has spread far beyond the Indian subcontinent to where it is native, and it is considered an invasive species. The species *Acacia confusa*, known as the rainbow tree, has one of the highest DMT concentrations yet reported in a plant; with the highest concentrations occurring in the root bark. As mentioned by Luken et al.[11] it has become invasive on Hawaii, supplanting the native Acacia, on an island with a long history of ecological disturbance that was ignited following the arrival of Man to the islands and continues to unfold. Another DMT rich plant, *Mimosa tenuiflora*, has also spread outside its native range, and is considered an invasive species in the southern US. Elsewhere in the tropics, the ayahuasca vine *B. caapi* has been reported as a feral species, and has spread its tendrils of influence far beyond its Amazonian home. Thus its alliance with Mankind may have assured its long-term survival on the planet. Its increasing use by urban sects of the Santo Daime Church allows people a deep connection with Nature even while being largely cut off from it.

The plot thickens and the mystery deepens when looking at ayahuasca and the DMT-containing plants. The ayahuasca vine (*B. caapi*) is a rich source of monoamine oxidase inhibitors, in the form of beta-carboline compounds. Some of these closely resemble endogenous human compounds such as pinoline. At high doses *B. caapi* can induce psychedelic effects. However it is the synergy with the DMT-containing plants chacruna (*Psychotria viridis*) and chaliponga (*Diplopterys cabrerana*) where an amazing feat of plant alchemy takes place. The MAOIs present in the vine allow DMT, that would otherwise be rapidly broken down by the enzymes they inhibit, to pass into the blood stream and cross the blood-brain barrier. Furthermore, one of the most ancient of human technologies, fire, is employed for cooking up the brews to release the active alkaloids from the plant material and prepare this as a tea for consumption.

The standard anthropological theory of how the indigenous people in Amazonia discovered the powerful synergistic visionary effects when combining the plants is that it was via trial and error of different species they encountered in their environment. This however is not a view shared by the people in question, claiming that their knowledge came directly from 'the plant teachers' as mentioned by Luna.[12] Amazonia is one of the most biodiverse parts of the world, with many thousands of plant species, and many different tribes across Amazonia have made this discovery, suggesting that there may be something more than trial and error at work. Ayahuasca itself has been seen as an agent that transcends this system of trial and error. According to Kaxinawá legend, it was an ayahuasca experience that bestowed upon them knowledge of the kambo medicine. A shaman was attempting to heal his tribe and he had exhausted other remedies from the forest that were available to him. So he took ayahuasca as a last resort to seek advice on how to help his people. The ayahuasca showed him a vision of the monkey tree frog (*Phyllomedusa bicolor*) and gave him advice on how to use its defensive skin secretions to heal. While a distinct tree frog in appearance, this is one of many tree frog species that inhabits Amazonia.

DMT is a simple molecule closely related to serotonin and derived from the amino acid tryptophan which is very widespread and abundant in the natural world and the compound has been detected in a number of species, including humans, and appears to be highly abundant and widespread in the botanical realm. Interestingly, the precise role it plays in humans, and its biological significance in other species, remains unclear. It seems that the enzymes responsible for its synthesis are ancient and shared by many different species, so DMT can act as a common biochemical denominator that can transcend species barriers across the biosphere. This emphasises on a tangible, biochemical level that we are all interconnected and interrelated. With the MAOI's and DMT, plants have found a way to powerfully hack into the nervous systems of other species. DMT has recently been found to be present in the pineal glands of live rats, as reported by Barker et al.,[13] and there may also be evidence for its in situ synthesis there. The pineal gland is an extremely ancient evolutionary development in vertebrate brains, and is present in all but the most primitive vertebrates and a few evolutionary exceptions. The rodent and primate lineages only parted on the evolutionary tree of life around 70 million years ago, which in terms of evolutionary time on this planet, all of 3.7 billion years, isn't long. Rodents make excellent model animals due to the profound biochemical and physiological similarities in which their cells function compared to us. Thus DMT is very likely present in us and many other species, although its physiological role remains a mystery.

The psychedelic plants, fungi and animals that are a part of the biosphere may have some extremely valuable lessons and insights to teach us relating to life on this planet, and our species would be foolish to disregard these fascinating species. We are currently in the midst of the sixth global mass extinction, which is down purely to our actions on the biosphere. With the destruction of the natural world and the rainforest we are continuously losing species, some of which may have highly valuable properties, but shall be lost forever. Man would be wise to broaden its cognitive horizons and pursue any avenues that allow for a deeper, more comprehensive, all-encompassing view of the natural world, and our part in it. An enhanced connection to life also has benefits that go both ways; it is not just good for the Earth, it directly benefits our species too, and we'd be foolish to dismiss this core teaching of the psychedelic experience hastily. The rise of depression and anxiety conditions in the Western world may be symptoms of our increasing societal disconnect with the natural world, as well as our fellow humans, and this takes a substantial and increasing personal and economic toll every year. Psychedelic experiences have the power to cut through the superficial materialistic and consumerist mindset in a powerful way and reconnect us with the pulsing heart that is the mystery of nature of which we are all a part. As Dennis McKenna felt he was told by the ayahuasca vine on his first experience with the plant: 'You monkeys only think you're running things'. We could likely all benefit from being humbled in this manner. Human exploration by way of these transformative agents may be highly valuable in instilling these values in us, and this will be of benefit to ourselves, all life, and our long-term future on this planet.

References:

1. Krippner, S., Luke, D. 'Psychedelics and Species Connectedness'. In *Bulletin: Psychedelics and Ecology*. Brown, D.J. (ed). MAPS. 2009 19(1):12–15.

2. Doblin, R., Burge, B. 'Manifesting Minds: A Review of Psychedelics'. In *Science, Medicine, Sex, and Spirituality*. North Atlantic Books. 2014.

3. Rome, A. '"Give Earth a Chance": The Environmental Movement and the Sixties'. *J Am Hist*. 2003 90(2):543–544.

4. Lerner, M., Lyvers, M. 'Values and beliefs of psychedelic drug users: a cross-cultural study'. *J Psychoactive Drugs*. 2006 38:143–147.

5. Studerus, E., Kometer, M., Hasler, F., Vollenweider, F.X. 'Acute, subacute and long-term subjective effects of psilocybin in healthy humans: a pooled analysis of experimental studies'. *J Psychopharmacol*. 2011 25:1434–1452.

6. Maclean, K.A., Johnson, M.W., Griffiths, R.R. 'Mystical experiences occasioned by the hallucinogen psilocybin lead to increases in the personality domain of openness'. *J Psychopharmacol* (Oxford). 2011 25(11):1453–1461.

7. Smith, C.S. 'Albert Hofmann, the Father of LSD, Dies at 102'. *The New York Times*. April 30, 2008. Retrieved November 1, 2014.

8. Schroll, M.A., Rothenberg, D. 'Psychedelics and the Deep Ecology Movement: A Conversation with Arne Naess'. In *Bulletin: Psychedelics and Ecology*. Brown, D.J. (ed). MAPS. 2009 19(1):41–43.

9. Geml, J., Laursen, G.A., O'Neill, K., Nusbaum, C., Taylor, D.L. 'Beringian origins and cryptic speciation events in the fly agaric (Amanita muscaria)'. *Mol Ecol.* 2006 15:225–239.

10. Lee, M.A. *Smoke Signals: A Social History of Marijuana—Medical, Recreational and Scientific.* Simon and Schuster. 2013. 143.

11. Luken, J.O., Thieret, J.W. 'Amur honeysuckle, its fall from grace'. *Bioscience.* 1996 4:18–24.

12. Luna, L.E. 'The concept of plants as teachers among four mestizo shamans of Iquitos, northeast Peru.' *J Ethnopharmacol.* 1984 11:135–156.

13. Barker, S.A., Borjigin, J., Lomnicka, I., Strassman, R. 'LC/MS/MS analysis of the endogenous dimethyltryptamine hallucinogens, their precursors, and major metabolites in rat pineal microdialysate'. *Biomed Chromatogr.* 2013 27,(12):1690–1700.

PSYCHEDELICS IN THE ANTHROPOCENE

ALLAN BADINER

There is new enthusiasm for experience with psychedelics as tools for our evolution. Buddhism and psychedelic exploration share a common concern: the liberation of the mind. Could psychedelics, supported by an ancient system of ethics, become regarded as a cultural and ecological imperative for our survival? Is it fair to ask what else can offer the kind of mental evolution, political and social change with the rapidity required by our degenerating ecosystem?

Popularised by Nobel Laureate chemist Paul Crutzen, the term Anthropocene describes the new geologic epoch that the Earth has moved into since the stability of the planetary system was disrupted by human industrial activity, mainly the burning of fossil fuels for energy. As Crutzen observed, 'For the first time in Earth's history, its future is being determined by both the conscious and unconscious actions of Homo sapiens.'

'When humans look back,' according to Professor Will Steffen of the Australian National University, 'the Anthropocene will probably represent one of the six biggest extinctions in our planet's history.'

Affecting every climatic region of the Earth, the concentration of carbon in the atmosphere is dramatically intensifying, and global average temperatures continue to increase significantly. We are all familiar with the effects: melting ice caps, and global weather patterns fluctuating frequently between extremes. Global bodies meet periodically to discuss the problem, but to date no binding commitments to reduce carbon emissions have resulted.

The powerful petroleum industry that provides 80% of the global energy supply has a strong interest in maintaining the status quo regardless. The enormity of their profits and tens of billions of dollars of taxpayer subsidies in the US give them great power as measured in political influence, media manipulation, and the tendency to pull us into energy wars.

Yet, amidst what is essentially a slow motion ecological collapse, people remain in pursuit of greater fulfilment in their lives, seeking deeper spiritual truth and leaning about strategies for liberating themselves from suffering. Bound to be encountered on any journey to wisdom are Buddhism and psychedelics.

How does the issue of psychedelics find itself juxtaposed with the ancient wisdom tradition of Buddhism? It turns out that the same cast of characters (Alan Watts, Ram Dass, Jack Kerouac, Allen Ginsberg, etc.) that introduced America to psychedelics also brought us the first glimpse of the Buddha's teachings. Subsequently, nearly every Western-born Buddhist teacher admits to a previous phase in which they experimented with psychedelics.

Both in Buddhist and psychedelic experience, great value is put on coming to terms with one's own mortality and impermanence, on comprehending reality directly rather than theoretically or abstractly, and on understanding the tenuous borders between self and others. We are witnessing a greater acknowledgement of psychedelic use in a spiritual context, and a flowering of books and magazine stories evidence a sharp rise in intellectual interest. All of this is tantamount to a revolution in our understanding of the mind itself, and in the ways that psychedelic interventions may result in evolutionary mental advancement.

Meanwhile, emblematic of our time is that millions of people with the intent to reduce suffering, escape depression, or delusion are locked into taking expensive pharmaceutical drugs, all of which have formidable side effects, drug interactions and toxicity levels. Dennis

McKenna, PhD, estimates that about 10% of all teens and adults in America are on medications such as Lithium, Zopiclone, Citalopram, Ativan, Clonazepam, Seroquel, Resperidone, and Valium, just to name a few, most of which are now shown to promote the onset of Alzheimer's disease. Ironically, more people die every year from using prescription medicines than from illegal drugs.

Also presently in focus is the fact that many of the very plants and chemicals, such as LSD, psilocybin, MDMA and cannabis that were banned for the past 50 years, are now being studied as among the most promising interventions in a variety of difficult medical/mental conditions. For example, in 2014, the late Richard Rockefeller, MD, speaking at the Commonwealth Club in San Francisco, reported in an understated way the central finding of his studies: that MDMA has come closer than anything else to actually curing intractable PTSD.

Psilocybin, the active compound in magic mushrooms, is now known as much for the enduring improvement in the users' outlook on life as for vivid visuals and hallucinations. In one recent study, psilocybin dramatically and sustainably reduced the existential, end-of-life anxiety in dying cancer patients.

Thanks to studies by Dr Raphael Mechoulam, professor in the Department for Medicinal Chemistry at Hebrew University, we have discovered CBD, a molecule in cannabis that can have a powerful healing effect in the body for a multitude of conditions otherwise difficult to control or treat, such as Parkinson's disease, cancer, and neurological insults etc.

A dizzying resurgence of research into the therapeutic potential of controlled substances is now underway, and much more is warranted. After years of applications, the Federal government of the United States has finally approved a variety of clinical research studies, including most recently, a clinical trial using MDMA-assisted psychotherapy for anxiety associated with life-threatening illness. Most of the work with MDMA has been generated by the Multidisciplinary Association for Psychedelic Studies (MAPS), while the Heffter Research Institute has organised the majority of psilocybin studies.

Ralph Metzner PhD, one of the Harvard triumvirate with Timothy Leary and Ram Dass, once suggested that LSD was nothing less than a turning point in human evolution. Metzner asserted that Dr Hofmann's discovery of LSD shortly after the first nuclear bomb explosion was not a coincidence. He looked to LSD as a kind of divine antidote to the nuclear curse, and that humanity must pay heed to the psychedelic revelation if it is to alter its self-destructive course and avert a major catastrophe.

An important 'side effect' of these journeys appears to be an emergent awareness of one's immediate environment and attendant beings, as being sacred and inviolate. In the late 80s, once MDMA's empathogenic effects became more widely known, it was often joked that the most effective thing the environmental and social activists could do is put MDMA in the water supply. Can we reasonably expect yoga and meditation alone to be utilised at the level needed for evolutionary change?

Still, this only raises the question of a possible role that psychedelics have in the maturation of deep ecological intelligence and a sense of kinship with all life. It is arguable that our only hope for surviving the man-made perils ahead is a rapid and thorough awakening of this kind. The bodhisattva path may become a new archetype for psychedelically driven planetary activism.

Veneration for the induced visionary experience has roots in virtually every culture on earth, and one could argue that the use of visionary plants has been seminal to the development of civilisation. Two of the most pervasive and influential cultures the planet has ever seen, that of Hellenistic Greece and Aryan India, contained at their very core inspirations derived from the ingestion of psychedelic concoctions.

Dr Stanley Krippner, a leading parapsychologist, points out that while psychedelic substances have been used very wisely in many primitive cultures for spiritual and healing purposes, 'Our culture doesn't have this framework. We don't have the closeness to God, the closeness to nature, or the shamanistic outlook. We've lost all that.' This is perhaps where Buddhism comes in with an ethic of compassion and time-tested teachings that promote awareness, kindness, and self-development.

It is in this context that writer Robert Thurman, the first American to be ordained a Tibetan Monk by the Dalai Lama, and who has never been a psychedelic enthusiast, told a crowd of 300 at Burning Man in 2014 that when one considers the magnitude of the challenges ahead, psychedelics that can rapidly develop our empathetic capacity and degree of gratefulness could be considered a skilful means provided they were used carefully. The fifth precept of Buddhism, Thurman added, was clearly referring to alcohol, which was seen—even in ancient times—as a huge social and health problem.

A new scientific study, published in the *Journal of Psychopharmacology*, looked at 190,000 respondents from 2008 to 2012 and found that the classic psychedelics were not associated with adverse mental health outcomes. In addition, it found that people who had used LSD and psilocybin had lower lifetime rates of suicidal inclinations.

Along with recognition that some psychedelics may be a medicine not only for our bodies, minds, and spirit, but also for the health of the planet, they should nevertheless be approached with wisdom and caution, and with careful attention paid to set and setting.

It is becoming a less radical idea all the time, that what is good for the person is good for the planet. There is precious little time to reverse harmful habits and adopt healthy strategies for coping with the planetary crisis. Throughout his life, philosopher and psychedelic explorer Terence McKenna maintained that psychedelics give people the power to overcome habitual behaviours.

Psychedelic scholar Thomas Roberts has identified the stages of revolutionary change in this 'psychedelic renaissance' that many expect to result in long-term betterment. The velocity of this renaissance has it passing through all four stages simultaneously: The medical-neuroscientific stage, the spiritual-religious stage, the intellectual-artistic stage, and mind design stage.

This psychedelic revival is also evident in religious terms, with greater acknowledgement of psychedelic use in a spiritual context, for example the Native Americans have won a Supreme Court decision upholding their use of the shamanic plant peyote. There is a blossoming of books and websites that evidence the rise in intellectual interest (including my own: the new and revised edition of *Zig Zag Zen: Buddhism and Psychedelics,* coming out in May of this year). Most major religious traditions are in a dialogue with ayahuasca. Buddhist meditation teachers are regularly participating in Zen ayahuasca retreats in Peru and Ecuador.

On the other hand, as Huston Smith points out, 'While psychedelic use is all about altered states, Buddhism is all about altered traits, and one does not necessarily lead to the other.' When Ralph Metzner was asked by an interviewer if he thought that society had changed as a result of psychedelic use, he replied that it was impossible to say. 'I believe that the important thing is not drugs per se, but the notion and practice of expanding consciousness and taking many more perspectives into account in all situations... After all,' he added, 'Charles Manson used LSD, and look at what he did with it. What good was that?'

I fully understand the perspective that the use of psychoactive plants and Buddhist practice do not mix. In fact, this perspective is well represented in *Zig Zag Zen: Buddhism and Psychedelics,* prompting Brother David Steindl Rast, a Zen Benedictine monk, to say that the book 'shines by its fairness,' and that it 'squarely faces the Zig as well as the Zag... Zen at its best!' Compelling arguments against 'using while Buddhist' are offered by such highly regarded thinkers as Richard Baker Roshi, Robert Aitken Roshi, Brad Warner, and others.

But no one is waiting for a book to give permission to use psychedelics. The interest in, and use of, psychedelics for spiritual purposes has always been with us—it is found in every spiritual tradition—and it is currently undergoing a renaissance. Psychedelics and Buddhist practice may have a significant relationship, but no hallucinatory experience can replace the daily discipline of meditation and ethical practice. It is also important to recognise that even as psychedelics have been known to facilitate very profound experiences, and have led, in some cases, to steady and disciplined meditative practice, this does not equate to the idea that psychedelics are necessarily a valid part of Buddhist practice.

Examining psychedelics and dharma teachings together, we may understand more deeply the essence of each. MAPS is working on a protocol that would investigate the use of psychedelics in the midst of a 7–10 day Zen meditation retreat. This study would be conducted with Dr Franz Vollenweider, Professor of Psychiatry in the School of Medicine, University of Zürich, and a director at the Heffter Institute. Roland Griffiths, a professor of psychiatry and behavioural sciences at Johns Hopkins, is leading new research into the use of psilocybin among long-term meditators.

While the question of how Buddhism and psychedelics relate is not easily answered, science may prove to be the mediating field within which they meet with clarity and transparency going into the future. As noted by Christian Schwägerl, 'Human creativity, community spirit and conscious thought can lead to changes that might make our species look back at current behavior as sheer ecological barbarism.' Perhaps our salvation is recognising that in the Anthropocene, humans must own their power, work collaboratively, and take responsibility for changing our self-destructive behaviour that threatens all life.

Sources:

Schwägerl, C. The Anthropocene: *The Human Era and How It Shapes Our Planet*. Renner Jones, L. (trans). Synergetic Press. 2014.

Richardson, K., Steffen, W. *Climate Change: Global Risks, Challenges and Decisions*. Cambridge University Press. 2014.

Colgan, J. *Petro-Aggression: When Oil Causes War*. Cambridge University Press. 2013.

Wasson, G. *Persephone's Quest: Entheogens and the Origins of Religion*. Yale University Press. 1992.

Walsh, R., Grob, C.S. *Higher Wisdom: Eminent Elders Explore the Continuing Impact of Psychedelics*. State University of New York Press. 2005.

Merz, B. 'Benzodiazepine Use May Raise Risk of Alzheimer's Disease'. Harvard Health Blog. Harvard Medical School. September 10, 2014.

Leary, T. *The Politics of Ecstasy*. Ronin Publishing. 1998.

Campos, Don J. *The Shaman & Ayahuasca: Journeys To Sacred Realms*. Divine Arts. 2011.

'Ayahuasca, Plant Dieta & Buddhist Meditation Retreat'. <http://www.sacred-spiritjourneys.com/sacred-journey-peru---ayahuasca.html>

Hayes, C. *Tripping: An Anthology of True-Life Psychedelic Adventures*. Penguin Compass. 2000.

Lee, M.A. *Acid Dreams: The Complete Social History of LSD: The CIA, the Sixties, and Beyond*. Grove Press. 1994.

Krebs, Teri Suzanne. 'Psychedelics not linked to mental health problems or suicidal behavior: A population study'. *Journal of Psychopharmacology*. Department of Neuroscience, Norwegian University of Science and Technology, Trondheim, N-7489, Norway. Email: krebs@ntnu.no, <http://jop.sagepub.com/content/29/3/270>

Roberts, T.B. 'How Psychedelics Might Transform the Human Mind and Lead Humanity

Towards Intellectual and Artistic Heights. A four-stage preview'. AlterNet. February 26, 2015 <http://www2.alternet.org/drugs/psychedelic-renaissance-here-eternity>

RISKS AND HARMS ON PSYCHEDELICS

DEALING WITH POWERFUL, EMOTIONALLY INTENSE EXPERIENCES IN THE CONTEXT OF PSYCHOLYTIC THERAPY

FRIEDERIKE MECKEL FISCHER

Would you really enter an airplane, without knowing the heights you are climbing, where you are going to land and what to expect in the new country? Would you go without any luggage, without any companion, blindfolded?

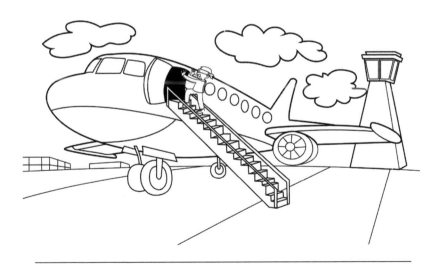

Would you assume that this trip must carry you into nirvana? Would you fly without your seat belt fastened? How will you react, when the plane starts shaking and swaying? What will happen, when things become very uncomfortable, when you get frightened? When you finally are convinced that the plane is crashing and your blood freezes?

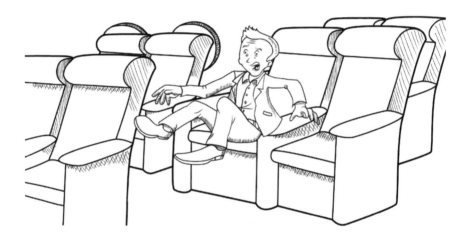

On whom will you put the blame for this, after an uneasy landing? The plane? The storm? The guy who sold you the ticket? And how will you name this in the end? A bad trip?

PSYCHEDELIC EXPERIENCES

There are those which bring you close to enlightenment—where you are in an oceanic state of being, in unity with yourself and the universe, in pure consciousness, love and peace.

There are those which bring you close to disintegration, where you feel disconnected from yourself and the world, in the void, in pure fear, horror and mortal agony. There are many other experiences in between. These are the most common ones. Experiences associated with 'positive feelings' are preferred and popularly called 'good trips'. Those associated with 'negative feelings' are called 'bad trips'.

I am invited here as a therapist which has worked with LSD, MDMA, 2CB and Psilocybin.

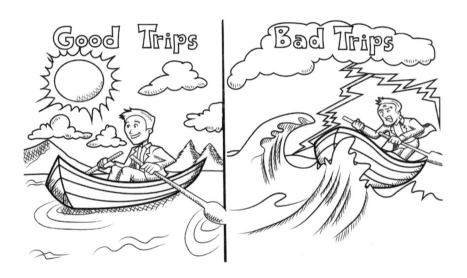

In this context, I will focus today on the difficult experiences and I will talk about:

DEALING WITH POWERFUL, DIFFICULT, EMOTIONALLY INTENSE EXPERIENCES IN THE CONTEXT OF PSYCHOLYTIC THERAPY

I will outline why these experiences are especially welcome in psycholytic therapy and how they are converted into lasting corrective new experiences and will lead to the authentic personality.

I will first explain some theoretical basics. I will talk about:

- Function of the substances.
- Conscious and unconscious memories of a person, where they are stored and their variety in appearing in psycholytic sessions.
- Phenomenon of projection.
- Importance of the triad of dose, set and setting.
- Psycholytic therapy and its purpose.
- Emergence of difficult life events, the work-through and tools.
- Principles of resolving traumatising events.
- Corrective new experiences.
- Integration steps.

FUNCTION OF PSYCHOACTIVE SUBSTANCES

The substances LSD, 2CB and psilocybin do not have any pharmacological potential of their own, which means they are not specific for any purpose, like Aspirin might be for a headache. The scientific world agrees that using them is not dangerous to health.

MDMA has some contraindications and some restrictions, which should be known: High blood pressure, asthma medication, beta blockers, antidepressants or HIV-medication.

Psychoactive substances do not create feelings. They function like catalysts for psychic and mental insights that can lead to change in life. They expand the conscious awareness. They allow any event in a person's biography—noticed, heard, seen, felt, smelled—liked or disliked at the time of their occurrence, to surface. They are door openers to the unconscious. They allow any event, from procreation to this very day, to emerge. These events—forgotten, repressed or dissociated—emerge with their associated perceptions, feelings and body sensations.

Psychoactive substances mirror the person's own life. The substances only excavate what is stored. One only perceives their very own inside. Psychoactive substances facilitate encountering oneself in all respects.

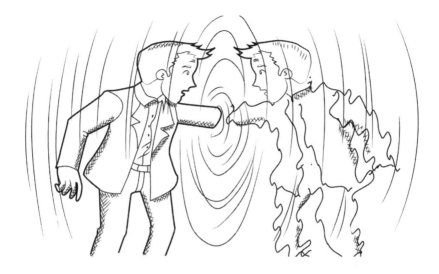

POWERFUL EXPERIENCES IN REAL LIFE

Powerful experiences are emotionally intense experiences with an impact. They first happen in real life. The bad trip in a later session is only the replay of a former reality, showing up in a condensed, possibly alienated form. When the event happened first, it was unconsciously stored as perceived: horrifying, threatening, tied together with its accompanying feelings. Naturally the same happens with joyous events: the inner state of the moment is the crucial criterion, which will be remembered.

The earlier intense impacts take place, the more they determine the perception of the world. They are hidden, secret guides, steering the actions and reactions of a person. They determine self-perception, like: 'I am stupid'. They turn into survival concepts, like 'I have to perform, to be loved'. They manifest as attitudes, belief-systems. They may lead to dysfunctional neurotic behaviour, compulsive patterns or personality disorders and thus become the source of difficulties in relationships.

Repressed or dissociated, they are not accessible to memory any more. Intense experiences can happen at any time. You fall in love the first time, the butterfly feelings in your stomach are engraved as stored patterns and become your future when judging a love-relationship.

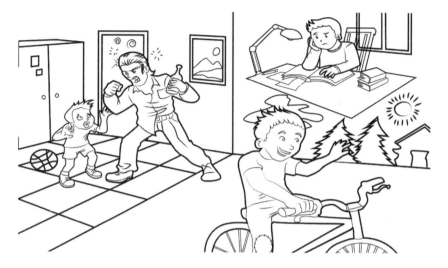

The ability to love and relate as trustworthy is already predetermined by the quality of binding and bonding with mother and father, the first shaping encounter with relationship.

You experience a traffic accident, you survive, your best friend dies. The frozen shock will be stored, conscious and unconsciously—depending on the impact, the event might even be dissociated.

EMERGENCE OF EXPERIENCES

Psychoactive substances only convey and reveal a person's own psychic material. This can manifest itself on a session through thoughts, convincing insights, images, feelings, body sensations, and many other different states of being.

Contents of experiences may appear clearly and may easily be understood as one's own biographical scenes. But they may also show up metaphorically through strange images, so that they need to be decrypted. Life events of our ancestors may appear as pictures or scenes, and can be interpreted as epigenetic phenomena.

Contents of experiences may appear repeatedly, with vague feelings, strange body-sensations, blurred images. These often point to very early formative, preverbal, intrauterine or perinatal experiences or to dissociated biographical events.

They too need to be decoded, put into words. Sometimes this is possible already in the session, sometimes only afterwards. All of these need to be identified, worked through and assigned to the underlying event.

Contents of stress-associated experiences can show in the form of body reactions, such as shaking, trembling or freezing. The associated difficult feelings can emerge at the same time, or later in another session.

Dissociation mostly first shows up as confusion, agitation, disconnectedness or nonspecific unease. The client will report that nothing is happening or he complains to have received an ineffective low dose. It is necessary to stay with the client, help discover the causal event on one hand and reconnect carefully with the associated feelings on the other hand, before reliving the experience and then letting it go.

Psychedelic experiences open the unconscious, stir up all kinds of memories and thus mirror the inside of a person. To put it in one sentence: In good times and in bad times: All you meet is you.

PHENOMENON OF PROJECTION

Unfortunately it is not common knowledge that the contents of experiences only belong to the person herself.

Not being aware of this, a client will assume that images or feelings exist outside of him and come from the outside. He will deny their existence within himself and attribute them to others. This is called projection.

Without guidance to how to work with a substance, he will react on upcoming emotionally difficult issues the same way as initially and thus stumble into a retraumatisation.

Sensations like fear, anxiety, sad or painful memories, body pain or nausea are generally unwelcome. Called 'negative feelings', they will be fought off and rejected. This worsens the already bad condition.

Images, read as coming from the outside, are named hallucinations, 'seeing something that is not there'. When they are scary, people become afraid of their own inner life.

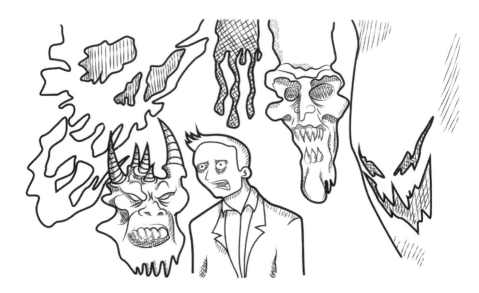

Every person taking a psychoactive substance needs to be familiar with the phenomenon of projection and should learn not to react, especially to unpleasant feelings and images. Otherwise, his venture can turn into what is called a 'bad trip'. **Among other preconditions, a really good bad trip starts out of projection.**

BASE FOR PSYCHOLYTIC THERAPY: DOSE, SET AND SETTING

The dose of a known substance should match exactly to the client's needs. His previous experiences and his intention should be considered. In general the principle of Paracelsus applies: 'the dose makes the poison', especially with LSD and psylocybin. Everything concerning the client is called set. The client must be prepared; he must have an intention and needs to feel safe.

Everything concerning the therapist is called setting. His professionality and the ambience he offers must be up to the task. The fulfilled conditions of dose, set and setting, are the 'controlled setting', the centrepiece of psycholytical therapy.

PSYCHOLYTIC THERAPY

The use of psychoactive substances enables access to the unconscious, elucidation of the conscious, contact with the collective knowledge and the mystical. It paves the way to integration of what has been perceived—frightening or blissful—and in the end to the authentic self.

PURPOSE OF PSYCHOLYTIC THERAPY

The main goal is a change in life for the better: Integration through work-up of any kind of psychic disorders, harms, insults, painful experiences, traumatising events and their aftereffects, like neurosis and the Post Traumatic Stress Disorder. It is the reintegration of dissociated parts of the personality. In this regard, it does not differ much from conventional therapy.

It is also about climbing the steep ladder of self-knowledge from the valley of unconscious disturbances to becoming aware of one's own inherent qualities, and it is about seeking a way to move towards a sustainable change in the values of life. This is the moment to mention the ongoing studies with MDMA on Post Traumatic Stress Disorders (PTSD) all over the world and to thank all participants.

EMERGENCE OF DIFFICULT LIFE
EVENTS IS MOST WELCOME

Since real life 'bad trips' control us secretly, and since the substances give access to their not consciously known psychic impact, we welcome difficult emotionally intense experiences to emerge. The goal for the client is to gain a deep understanding of and agreement with the past situation, its participants and the circumstances and thus reach a different point of view. Moreover many a client may get an understanding of the roots of his addiction.

EMERGENCE OF DIFFICULT LIFE EVENTS IS INTENDED

In our controlled setting a client would direct his intention towards a bad experience from the past and face it. Initially he stops fighting. He bids the dragon to stop being dangerous. He looks deep into the dragon's eyes. For the first time in life, they see and recognise each other.

The dragon is taken by surprise; when the hero touches him fearlessly and as a friend, his evil power diminishes. The touch tames the dragon and transformation takes place. The chain that has tied the two together dissolves, and the dragon transmutes into the enormous force of the client, which had been frozen by fear.

Past experiences sometimes *occur spontaneously*. Then they would be treated the same way.

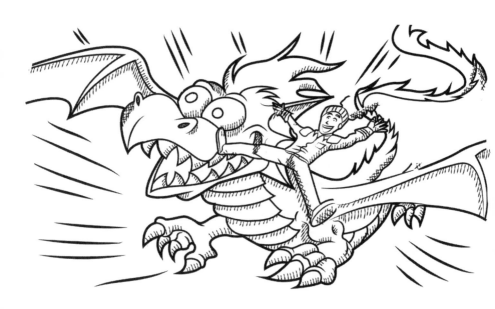

TOOLS

The emerging material determines the tool.

- One tool is the client's own observing of his process, memorising the answers and insights.
- One tool is the therapist. His talking or listening, answering or asking questions. His guiding through moving moments, with or without body contact or words.
- Modified family-constellation-work shows the hidden dynamics of a system, epigenetic or transgenerational phenomena.
- Life bodywork in the 'as-if-now-modus', the work-through for traumatising events.
- There is the group-interaction to represent the world and to provide support.
- Naturally there is music, to guide through emotions.

Not only difficult experiences must emerge completely. For final integration they have to be worked through, sometimes a couple of times. They must be understood and agreed to on body, mind and soul level.

PRINCIPLES OF RESOLVING TRAUMATISING EVENTS

The traumatising event links with the perception, reaction, the associated feelings and sensations of the moment. Whenever a trigger is perceived, unconscious associations arise and the system reacts in its specific way. To resolve, the link between the identified traumatic event and the associated emotions must be cut.

The 'cutting' needs an environment of trust. For reliving the event, the client's 'grown-up self' part stays in contact with the therapist, the other part, the 'hurt-child', remains in contact with its feelings and perceptions.

By reliving and acknowledging the event to be over, the cut is done. This might be expressed by sentences like: 'This is how it was. It is history now. I can memorise it without being carried away.' To achieve

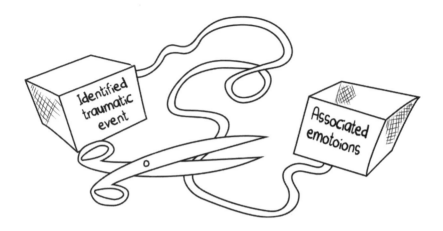

a sustainable change in life after this process, the client now must develop new patterns, exercise them and reorganise his daily life.

CORRECTIVE NEW EXPERIENCES

Corrective new experiences can arise from insights that you are able to feel and to love, that you are not alone and that you are a lovable person yourself.

Another important healing experience is to develop the courage to open up and find out, not to be hurt by daring to do this, or even by making friends.

INTEGRATION STEPS

Complete integration means reaching a grown-up state of being.

- The first step in the session itself is to rationally and emotionally take in the event, reliving the emotions and cutting the emotional link between the two.
- Expressing the process in sharing, writing a protocol and a therapeutic meeting in between sessions represent the meta-level. These are the second, third and fourth steps on the integration ladder.

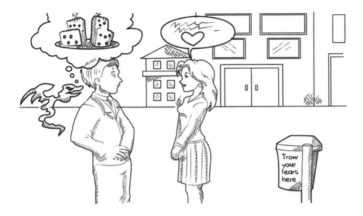

- The fifth step is attentiveness in daily life to detect traces of old reactions and having the courage to change them.
- When difficult feelings transmute into serenity, they become an integrated part of personality. This is the sixth step.

Generally speaking, pscholytic therapy helps with integrating the shadows, leading to fewer projections in everyday life. Bad trips in life result in suffering and fighting in daily life. To bring this to an end, we want to resolve them in psycholytic therapy.

The door openers to the unconscious facilitate their lively emergence. The substances, the person's own work through, and the tools help dissolve and let corrective new experiences happen—pathways to the authentic personality.

Thus, **stumbling stones that bad trips are made of will turn into stepping-stones.**

ONE LAST WORD

I am sure that you are people who prefer meaningful journeys instead of recreational trips. You will carefully choose a destination, route and the best, not the cheapest airline. You will pack the suitcase functionally and even prepare yourself for the case that in spite of all your preparations the weather might turn stormy. Maybe you like to take your partner along or even take a tour guide. I suppose you embark on this journey for the sake of your inner development.

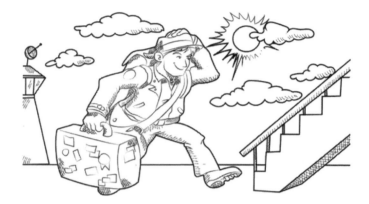

SPECIAL FEATURES OF SPECIAL K

APPLICATIONS FOR PAIN AND DEPRESSION TREATMENTS

THARCILA CHAVES

IT HURTS

The International Association for the Study of Pain defines pain as an unpleasant sensory and emotional experience associated with actual or potential tissue damage, or described in terms of such damage.[1] The mechanisms by which tissue injuries produce a state of pain represent one of the most intensely investigated areas in the biomedical sciences over several years.[2]

Glutamate, the major excitatory neurotransmitter in the brain and spinal cord, exerts its postsynaptic effects via a diverse set of membrane receptors. Of these, NMDA receptors have received particular attention because of their crucial roles in excitatory synaptic transmission, plasticity and neurodegeneration in the central nervous system.[2]

Ketamine, also known as 'special K', increases the presynaptic release of glutamate, resulting in higher extracellular levels of glutamate by a combination of disinhibition of the neurotransmitter gamma-aminobutyric acid (GABA) and blockage of the NMDA receptors at the phencyclidine site within the ion channel.[5] This increase in extracellular glutamate release favours co-expressed α-amino-3-hydroxy-5-methyl-4-isoxazolepropionic acid (AMPA), resulting in an increased glutamatergic throughput of AMPA relative to NMDA.[5]

Ketamine is a well-known human anaesthetic, with analgesic effects that may be used to treat pain in a range of disorders.[6] In the field of pain management, there is ample experience with oral as well as intravenous applications of ketamine. Indications for ketamine include neuropathic pain of various origins, complex regional pain syndrome, cancer pain, orofacial pain and phantom limb pain.

There is considerable evidence that pain associated with peripheral tissue or nerve injury involves activation of NMDA receptors.[7] Consistent with this, NMDA receptor antagonists have been shown to effectively alleviate pain-related behaviour.[8-23] However, the use of NMDA receptor antagonists can often be limited by serious side effects, such as memory impairment, psychotomimetic effects, ataxia and motor incoordination.[2]

SOME RELIEF

Ketamine is a non-selective NMDA receptors antagonist, and due to the presence of a chiral centre, it has 2 enantiomers (FIGURE 1): S-ketamine and R-ketamine. The S-enantiomer is marketed in Europe (trade name 'ketanest'); the rest of the world makes use of the racemic mixture (trade name 'ketalar').[24]

Ketamine is effective in acute and chronic pain with important differences in pharmacodynamics between these pain states. Analgesia induced by ketamine for acute pain relief is driven by the drug's pharmacokinetics with a short half-life of effect (1 to 10 minutes) and displays an immediate loss of analgesia upon the termination of ketamine administration. On the other hand, analgesia for neuropathic pain relief is best induced via a long-term infusion, with treatments lasting days (even weeks) rather than hours, making the analgesia persist for days and weeks beyond the exposure time (half-life for effect: 10 to 11 days).[24]

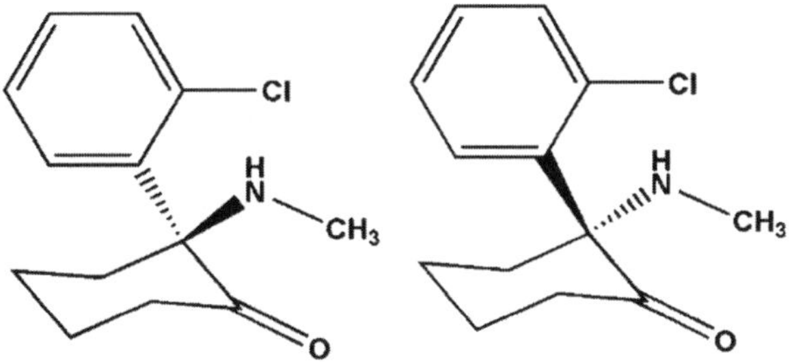

R-(–)- ketamine   S-(+)- ketamine

FIGURE 1: Ketamine's chirality

Ketamine metabolism happens in the liver through the cytochrome P450 enzyme system. Ketamine metabolites include norketamine (80%), hydroxynorketamine (15%) and hydroxyketamine (5%). In humans, these metabolites have a limited contribution to ketamine effect. The N-demethylation into norketamine is the major metabolic pathway. At clinical concentrations, N-demethylation is catalysed by CYP3A4 and CYP2B6. All metabolites undergo glucuronidation, followed by elimination via kidneys and liver, with 10 to 20% of ketamine being excreted unchanged.[25, 26]

The most common side effects of intravenous ketamine are psychotomimetic effects and dissociative symptoms,[27] such as confusion, dizziness, euphoria, elevated blood pressure and increased libido, although all of these usually dissipate within two hours of intravenous (IV) infusion.[28, 29] The increased blood pressure can be managed with the concomitant use of a benzodiazepine.[10, 13]

Another concern with ketamine is its abuse potential, which has been demonstrated in both animals and humans.[30, 31] Ketamine has been used recreationally since the 1960s. The so-called 'side effects' (hallucinations and dissociative experiences) might be perceived as 'desired effects' by people with psychonautic purposes.

An important reason to focus on NMDA receptor antagonists is that current treatment paradigms based on antidepressants, antiepileptics, slow-release opioid and local treatment (e.g. lidocaine or capsaicine patch) are only effective in 30% of patients. Therefore, there is the urgent need for an additional treatment that will cover a larger percentage of patients.[24]

The most effective ketamine treatment is by IV infusion. This in-house therapy is expensive and there is the need for at home ketamine treatment possibilities. Currently this is possible, for example, by using oral or nasal ketamine. However, due to a low bioavailability the probability of long-term success is restricted. Concerning bioavailability, it should be noted that this is only between 17%[32] and 23%[33] in oral administration, because of its extensive first-pass metabolism.[32] Intranasally, ketamine has a bioavailability of 45%.[34] Furthermore, the current ketamine solution is bitter, lowering patient compliance and adherence to therapy. Niesters and Dahan (2012) recommend that new modes of administration need to be developed. The expectation is that new modes of administration should be well accepted and should have a high bioavailability.[24]

Therefore, extensive knowledge on the pharmacokinetics and pharmacodynamics of ketamine, its enantiomers and its metabolites is required, so that careful treatment of the patient is possible, aimed at optimal pain relief combined with minimal side effects.

BUT LIFE STILL SUCKS

Depression is a very common mental disorder. Globally, more than 350 million people of all ages suffer from depression. It is the leading cause of disability and economic burden worldwide.[35] Although there are medications that alleviate depressive symptoms, these have serious limitations. Most notably, available treatments require weeks or months to produce a therapeutic response, and only about one-third of patients respond to the first medication prescribed.[36, 37]

Hallucinogenic drugs produce alterations in consciousness, perception, thought and emotion, and have been used recreationally and entheogenically for millennia. So-called 'classical' psychedelic drugs such as lysergic acid diethylamide (LSD), psilocybin, dimethyltryptamine (DMT) and mescaline are thought to exert their effects through agonism at the 5-HT2A receptors. Dissociative hallucinogens including ketamine, phencyclidine (PCP) and dextromethorphan (DXM) act primarily as NMDA glutamate receptor antagonists.[38, 39] The subjective state of dissociation from the body commonly experienced after sufficiently high doses of ketamine is called the 'K-hole'.[40]

There has been growing interest in the observation that ketamine has a rapid positive effect on depressive symptoms. It has been more than a decade since ketamine, an anaesthetic medication, was first reported to have therapeutic effects in depression.[39] The fact that ketamine does not work through the conventional antidepressant monoaminergic targets of serotonin and noradrenaline has provoked excitement, and understanding its effects could provide novel insights into the pathophysiology of depression, opening up a new class of medications.[39] A study performed with rats has shown that the mechanisms underlying this effect involve the activation of the mammalian target of the rapamycin (mTOR) pathway and increases spine formation and synaptic transmission of neurons in the prefrontal cortex.[36]

Current pharmacologic treatments for depression consist of a usual armamentarium of more than 24 antidepressants with at least 7 different mechanisms of action.[37] Some studies state that the effects of ketamine occurred only at low doses, indicating that the antidepressant actions of ketamine need not be accompanied by psychedelic side effects.[38, 41] Ketamine is inexpensive and easy to administer. It also has a rapid onset of action and minimal side effects when used at subanaesthetic doses.[42]

Several studies demonstrate that ketamine is capable of inducing a robust antidepressant effect in patients with depression, which were previously refractory to standard treatment with oral antidepressants as well as electroconvulsive therapy.[38, 41, 43–49]

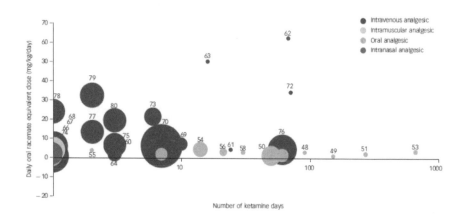

FIGURE 2: Overview of daily dose of ketamine for treating pain and number of ketamine days. Thirty-six studies about ketamine used for treating pain were included. The x-axis represents the number of ketamine days, which is different from the study duration (in some studies, only one or few doses were given during a long follow-up time). The size of the bubbles represents the sample size. The numbers close to the bubbles refer to the study identification, which can be found in the article published by Schoevers et al., 2016.[29]

A PILL FOR ALL PAINS?

With a team of researchers from the University of Groningen, I performed a literature review. It has been published in the *British Journal of Psychiatry*.[29] We searched PubMed with the terms 'ketamine', 'depression', 'chronic pain' and 'neuropathic pain'. It yielded 88 articles. All papers were scanned for dosages, amount of patients that received ketamine, number of ketamine days, results and side effects.

In the field of pain management, there is ample experience with utilising the oral as well as intravenous application method of ketamine. As in depression, the analgesic effect is believed to be based on antagonism of NMDA receptors.

FIGURE 2 gives an overview of the retrieved pain studies. The majority of them used the intravenous application of ketamine.

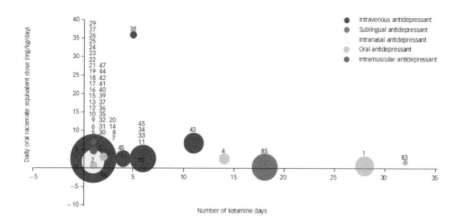

FIGURE 3: Overview of daily dose of ketamine for treating depression and number of ketamine days. Fifty-two studies about ketamine used to treat depression were included. The x-axis represents the number of ketamine days, which is different from the study duration (in some studies, only one or few doses were given during a long follow-up time). The size of the bubbles represents the sample size. The numbers close to the bubbles refer to the study identification, which can be found in the article published by Schoevers et al., 2016.[29]

The doses used in the pain studies differed from 0.1 to 62 mg/kg/day. It was not possible to establish a dose-response association, but the majority of pain studies describe ketamine as effective in reducing pain, even with low oral doses.

One study deserves a remark: the green bubble number 53.[50] In this study, oral ketamine was administered daily for 660 days at a dose of 3.4 mg/kg/day in one patient, with a significant improvement and non-severe side effects.

FIGURE 3 gives an overview of the retrieved depression studies. The majority of depression studies also used the intravenous application of ketamine. The most common dose was 0.5 mg/kg/day and other small doses, as we can see in the huge overlap of points close to the intersection of the x and y-axis.

The highest dose applied in a depression study was 36 mg/kg/day in 2 patients.[51] They had a very significant response with non-severe side effects—only a mild feeling of headiness was described.

From our literature review, we conclude that the doses used for depression are in the lower range compared to studies that investigated analgesic use. Also, ketamine as an antidepressant was generally given for shorter durations than ketamine as an analgesic.

We found no evidence for neurotoxicity caused by ketamine at therapeutic doses. Nevertheless, it is known that prolonged ketamine abuse has been associated with memory changes,[52] cognitive impairment,[27, 53] brain white matter changes[54] and reduced well-being.[27]

Also, inflammation and damage to the ureter and bladder are well documented in heavy ketamine users—around 80 mg/kg/day—which is more than 2 times higher than the highest dose found in a study where ketamine was used to treat depression.

Side-effects commonly mentioned were: dizziness, hallucinations, nausea, vomiting, drowsiness, confusion, light-headedness, headache, somnolence and anxiety. Adverse events did not persist after ketamine discontinuation. An interesting point is that the side effects were not reported as a burden in treatment maintenance.

THE AFTERGLOW

From our review, we conclude that there is sufficient scientific ground for future trials to incorporate longer treatment durations for depression based on the experience with ketamine in pain trials.

The reason why ketamine is still not officially approved as an analgesic and as an antidepressant might be controversial. There is vast scientific background showing that ketamine has manageable side effects, just as several drugs approved and being marketed right now do. The fact that ketamine is an old drug, that would not make a big profit for the pharmaceutical industry if marketed as an analgesic or antidepressant, should not be ignored.

Ketamine's afterglow, i.e. the rapid antidepressant effect of a single sub-anaesthetic intravenous dose of ketamine, which can last up to a month, is one of the most significant conceptual breakthroughs in the pharmacological treatment of depression. Ketamine has been proving to be a useful tool in treating depression and pain, and the fact that it is not being widely applied in current medicine is probably due to its recreational use (and the stigma surrounding it) more than the harm that it can cause. Although not official, the antidepressant and the analgesic uses of ketamine are already legitimate.

References:

1. International Association for the Study of Pain. IASP Taxonomy. Available at: http://www.iasp-pain.org/Education/Content.aspx?ItemNumber=1698&&navItemNumber=576#Pain. Accessed March 15th, 2016.

2. Petrenko, A.B., Yamakura, T., Baba, H., Shimoji, K. 'The role of N-methyl-D-aspartate (NMDA) receptors in pain: a review'. *Anesthesia & Analgesia.* 2003 97(4):1108–1116.

3. Moghaddam, B., Adams, B., Verma, A., Daly, D. 'Activation of glutamatergic neurotransmission by ketamine: a novel step in the pathway from NMDA receptor blockade to dopaminergic and cognitive disruptions associated with the prefrontal cortex'. *J Neurosci.* 15 April 1997 17(8):2921–2927.

4. Blonk, M.I., Koder, B.G., van den Bemt, P.M., Huygen, F.J. 'Use of oral ketamine in chronic pain management: a review'. *Eur J Pain May* 2010 14(5):466–472.

5. Doubell, T.P, Mannion, R., Woolf, C. 'The dorsal horn: state-dependent sensory processing, plasticity and the generation of pain'. *Textbook of Pain* 1999 4:165–181.

6. Elsewaisy, O., Slon, B., Monagle, J. 'Analgesic effect of subanesthetic intravenous ketamine in refractory neuropathic pain: a case report'. *Pain Med* June 2010 11(6):946–950.

7. Kang, J.G., Lee, C.J., Kim, T.H., Sim, W.S., Shin, B.S., Lee, S.H., et al. 'Analgesic effects of ketamine infusion therapy in Korean patients with neuropathic pain: A 2-week, open-label, uncontrolled study. *Curr Ther Res Clin Exp.* April 2010 71(2):93–104.

8. Schwartzman, R.J., Alexander, G.M., Grothusen, J.R., Paylor, T., Reichenberger, E., Perreault, M. 'Outpatient intravenous ketamine for the treatment of complex regional pain syndrome: a double-blind placebo controlled study'. *Pain.* 15 December 2009 147 (1–3):107–115.

9. Kvarnstrom, A., Karlsten, R., Quiding, H., Emanuelsson, B.M., Gordh, T. 'The effectiveness of intravenous ketamine and lidocaine on peripheral neuropathic pain'. *Acta Anaesthesiol Scand.* Aug 2003 47(7):868–877.

10. Mitchell, A.C. 'An unusual case of chronic neuropathic pain responds to an optimum frequency of intravenous ketamine infusions'. *J Pain Symptom Manage.* May 2001 21(5):443–446.

11. Mercadante, S., Arcuri, E., Tirelli, W., Casuccio, A. 'Analgesic effect of intravenous ketamine in cancer patients on morphine therapy: a randomized, controlled, double-blind, crossover, double-dose study'. *J Pain Symptom Manage.* October 2000 20(4):246–252.

12. Kaviani, N., Khademi, A., Ebtehaj, I., Mohammadi, Z. 'The effect of orally administered ketamine on requirement for anesthetics and postoperative pain in mandibular molar teeth with irreversible pulpitis'. *J Oral Sci.* December 2011 53(4):461–465.

13. Jennings, C.A., Bobb, B.T., Noreika, D.M., Coyne, P.J. 'Oral ketamine for sickle cell crisis pain refractory to opioids'. *J Pain Palliat Care Pharmacother.* June 2013 27(2):150–154.

14. Furuhashi-Yonaha, A., Iida, H., Asano, T., Takeda, T., Dohi, S. 'Short- and long-term efficacy of oral ketamine in eight chronic-pain patients'. *Can J Anesth.* October 2002 49(8):886–887.

15. Fitzgibbon, E.J., Hall, P., Schroder, C., Seely, J., Viola, R. 'Low dose ketamine as an analgesic adjuvant in difficult pain syndromes: a strategy for conversion from parenteral to oral ketamine'. *J Pain Symptom Manage.* February 2002 23(2):165–170.

16. Amin, P., Roeland, E., Atayee, R. 'Case report: efficacy and tolerability of ketamine in opioid-refractory cancer pain'. *J Pain Palliat Care Pharmacother.* September 2014 28(3):233–242.

17. Bredlau, A.L., McDermott, M.P., Adams, H.R., Dworkin, R.H., Venuto, C., Fisher, S.G., et al. 'Oral ketamine for children with chronic pain: a pilot phase 1 study'. *J Pediatr.* July 2013 163(1):194–200.e1.

18. Kannan, T.R., Saxena, A., Bhatnagar, S., Barry, A. 'Oral ketamine as an adjuvant to oral morphine for neuropathic pain in cancer patients'. *J Pain Symptom Manage.* January 2002 23(1.):60–65.

19. Vick, P.G., Lamer, T.J. 'Treatment of central post-stroke pain with oral ketamine'. *Pain.* May 2001 92(1–2):311–313.

20. Fisher, K., Hagen, N.A. 'Analgesic effect of oral ketamine in chronic neuropathic pain of spinal origin: a case report'. *J Pain Symptom Manage.* July 1999 18(1):61–66.

21. Nikolajsen, L., Hansen, P.O., Jensen, T.S. 'Oral ketamine therapy in the treatment of postamputation stump pain'. *Acta Anaesthesiol Scand.* March 1997 41(3):427–429.

22. Niesters, M., Dahan, A. 'Pharmacokinetic and pharmacodynamic considerations for NMDA receptor antagonists in the treatment of chronic neuropathic pain'. *Expert Opinion on Drug Metabolism & Toxicology.* 2012 8(11):1409–1417.

23. Hijazi, Y., Boulieu, R. 'Contribution of CYP3A4, CYP2B6, and CYP2C9 isoforms to N-demethylation of ketamine in human liver microsomes'. *Drug Metab Dispos.* July 2002 30(7):853–858.

24. Yanagihara, Y., Kariya, S., Ohtani, M., Uchino, K., Aoyama, T., Yamamura, Y., et al. 'Involvement of CYP2B6 in n-demethylation of ketamine in human liver microsomes'. *Drug Metab Dispos.* June 2001 29(6):887–890.

25. Morgan, C.J., Muetzelfeldt, L., Curran, H.V. 'Consequences of chronic ketamine self-administration upon neurocognitive function and psychological wellbeing: a 1-year longitudinal study'. *Addiction.* January 2010 105(1):121–133.

26. Liebrenz, M., Borgeat, A., Leisinger, R., Stohler, R. 'Intravenous ketamine therapy in a patient with a treatment-resistant major depression'. *Swiss Med Wkly.* 21 April 2007 137(15–16):234–236.

27. Schoevers, R.A., Chaves, T.V., Balukova, S.M., Rot, M.A., Kortekaas, R. 'Oral ketamine for the treatment of pain and treatment-resistant depression'. *The British Journal of Psychiatry*. The Royal College of Psychiatrists 2016 208(2):108–113.

28. Beardsley, P.M., Balster, R.L. 'Behavioral dependence upon phencyclidine and ketamine in the rat'. *J Pharmacol Exp Ther*. July 1987 242(1):203–211.

29. Klein, M., Calderon, S., Hayes, B. 'Abuse liability assessment of neuroprotectants'. *Ann N Y Acad Science*. 1999;890:515–525.

30. Clements, J.A., Nimmo, W.S., Grant, I.S. 'Bioavailability, pharmacokinetics, and analgesic activity of ketamine in humans'. *J Pharm Sci*. May 1982 71(5):539–542.

31. Chong, C., Schug, S., Page-Sharp, M., Ilett, K. 'Bioavailability of Ketamine After Oral or Sublingual Administration'. *Pain Medicine*. 2006 7(5):469–469.

32. Yanagihara, Y., Ohtani, M., Kariya, S., Uchino, K., Hiraishi, T., Ashizawa, N., et al. 'Plasma concentration profiles of ketamine and norketamine after administration of various ketamine preparations to healthy Japanese volunteers'. *Biopharm Drug Dispos*. January 2003 24(1):37–43.

33. World Health Organization. Depression —fact sheet number 369. 2012. Available at: http://www.who.int/mediacentre/factsheets/fs369/en/. Accessed July 7 2014.

34. Li, N., Lee, B., Liu, R.J., Banasr, M., Dwyer, J.M., Iwata, M., et al. 'mTOR-dependent synapse formation underlies the rapid antidepressant effects of NMDA antagonists'. *Science*. 20 August 2010 329(5994):959–964.

35. Stahl, S.M. *Stahl's Essential Psychopharmacology: neuroscientific basis and practical applications*. 3rd ed. New York: Cambridge University Press. 2008.

36. Salvadore, G., Singh, J.B. 'Ketamine as a fast acting antidepressant: current knowledge and open questions'. *CNS Neurosci Ther*. June 2013 19(6):428–436.

37. Caddy, C., Giaroli, G., White, T.P., Shergill, S.S., Tracy, D.K. 'Ketamine as the prototype glutamatergic antidepressant: pharmacodynamic actions, and a systematic review and meta-analysis of efficacy'. *Ther Adv Psychopharmacol*. April 2014 4(2):75–99.

38. Wikipedia. K-hole. Available at: http://en.wikipedia.org/wiki/K-hole. Accessed 11 June 2014.

39. Berman, R.M., Cappiello, A., Anand, A., Oren, D.A., Heninger, G.R., Charney, D.S., et al. 'Antidepressant effects of ketamine in depressed patients'. *Biol Psychiatry*. February 2000 15;47(4):351–354.

40. Irwin, S.A., Iglewicz, A. 'Oral ketamine for the rapid treatment of depression and anxiety in patients receiving hospice care'. *J Palliat Med*. July 2010 13(7):903–908.

41. Diamond, P.R., Farmery, A.D., Atkinson, S., Haldar, J., Williams, N., Cowen, P.J., et al. 'Ketamine infusions for treatment resistant depression: a series of 28 patients treated weekly or twice weekly in an ECT clinic'. *J Psychopharmacol*. 3 April 2014 28(6):536–544.

42. Lara, D.R., Bisol, L.W., Munari, L.R. 'Antidepressant, mood stabilizing and precognitive effects of very low dose sublingual ketamine in refractory unipolar and bipolar depression'. *Int J Neuropsychopharmacol*. October 2013 16(9):2111–2117.

43. Irwin, S.A., Iglewicz, A., Nelesen, R.A., Lo, J.Y., Carr, C.H., Romero, S.D., et al. 'Daily oral ketamine for the treatment of depression and anxiety in patients receiving hospice care: a 28-day open-label proof-of-concept trial'. *J Palliat Med*. August 2013 16(8):958-965.

44. Zarate Jr., C.A., Singh, J.B., Carlson, P.J., Brutsche, N.E., Ameli, R., Luckenbaugh, D.A., et al. 'A randomized trial of an N-methyl-D-aspartate antagonist in treatment-resistant major depression'. *Arch Gen Psychiatry.* August 2006 63(8):856–864.

45. Zarate Jr., C.A., Brutsche, N.E., Ibrahim, L., Franco-Chaves, J., Diazgranados, N., Cravchik, A., et al. 'Replication of ketamine's antidepressant efficacy in bipolar depression: a randomized controlled add-on trial'. *Biol Psychiatry.* 1 June 2012 71(11):939–946.

46. DiazGranados, N., Ibrahim, L.A., Brutsche, N.E., Ameli, R., Henter, I.D., Luckenbaugh, D.A., et al. 'Rapid resolution of suicidal ideation after a single infusion of an N-methyl-D-aspartate antagonist in patients with treatment-resistant major depressive disorder'. *J Clin Psychiatry.* December 2010 71(12):1605–1611.

47. Paslakis, G., Gilles, M., Meyer-Lindenberg, A., Deuschle, M. 'Oral administration of the NMDA receptor antagonist S-ketamine as add-on therapy of depression: a case series'. *Pharmacopsychiatry.* January 2010 43(1):33–35.

48. Villanueva-Perez, V.L., Cerda-Olmedo, G., Samper, J.M., Minguez, A., Monsalve, V., Bayona, M.J., et al. 'Oral ketamine for the treatment of type I complex regional pain syndrome'. *Pain Pract.* March 2007 7(1):39–43.

49. Correll, G.E., Futter, G.E. 'Two case studies of patients with major depressive disorder given low-dose (subanesthetic) ketamine infusions'. *Pain Med.* Jan-Feb 2006 7(1):92–95.

50. Freeman, T.P., Morgan, C.J., Pepper, F., Howes, O.D., Stone, J.M., Curran, H.V. 'Associative blocking to reward-predicting cues is attenuated in ketamine users but can be modulated by images associated with drug use'. *Psychopharmacology* (Berl) January 2013 225(1):41–50.

51. Morgan, C.J., Curran, H.V., Independent Scientific Committee on Drugs. 'Ketamine use: a review'. *Addiction.* January 2012 107(1):27–38.

52. Edward Roberts, R., Curran, H.V., Friston, K.J., Morgan, C.J.. 'Abnormalities in white matter microstructure associated with chronic ketamine use'. *Neuropsychopharmacology.* January 2014 39(2):329–338.

Statement of conflicts of interest
The author declares no conflicts of interest.

ACID MEDIUMSHIP: GOOSE AND CROW

JOHN CONSTABLE

This is the first time I've explicitly drawn attention to LSD as the catalyst for *The Southwark Mysteries*, although this multifaceted work is riddled with clues that it's rooted in a shamanistic experience—and is itself psychoactive, in the sense that recitation of the verses can evoke trance and transformative encounters with The Other. In the original poem that initiated the work, The Goose playfully asserts:

'... it must've given you a start
to find me so lysergic dear
when it comes to stealing hearts
and healing rifts between our hemispheres
there's no trick I wouldn't pull
to entice you
Over'ere.'[1]

This poem developed into a cycle of poems and contemporary Mystery Plays, and inspired a whole body of site-specific art and magic focused around protecting a graveyard in south London. Cross Bones was the outcasts' burial ground—for paupers, sex workers, anyone deemed unworthy of proper Christian burial. In medieval times, this was a fate worse than death, to be buried in unconsecrated ground, consigning the sinner's soul to Hell. *The Southwark Mysteries*, my Ur-text, seemed to spring, fully formed, from this desolate place. The complete work is published in my name, but in the preface I credit its true authors:

'The Southwark Mysteries were revealed by The Goose to John Crow at Cross Bones... on the night of the 23rd November 1996. My shamanic double had somehow raised the spirit of a medieval whore, licensed by a Bishop yet allegedly denied Christian burial:

For tonight in Hell
they are tolling the bell
for the Whore that lay at the Tabard,
and well we know
how the carrion crow
doth feast in our Cross Bones Graveyard.'[2]

The night I wrote these verses, I had no idea that Cross Bones really existed as a burial ground for paupers and, according to legend, 'Winchester Geese'—medieval sex workers, the 'Single Women' recorded by John Stow back in 1598.[3] That night, 23rd November 1996, I took what I've since referred to as 'an heroic dose' of LSD.

I was born a Goose of Southwark
by the Grace of Mary Overie,
whose Bishop gives me licence
to sin within The Liberty.
In Bankside stews and taverns
you can hear me honk right daintily,
as I unlock the hidden door,
unveil the Secret History.
I will dunk you in the river
and then reveal my Mystery.[4]

This is the first verse of the original poem which grew first into a cycle of poems, then Mystery Plays. The third part of the published work, the Glossolalia, is a compendium of esoteric lore. My editor had said: 'You can't call it a Glossary. Half the information was received from a spirit in a vision!' So... 'Glossolalia': a speaking in tongues.

Let's establish the set and setting in which this vision manifested. I'm a writer. I've spent much of my adult life writing for the theatre. As a playwright, it's my job to cultivate voices, to create characters that have an autonomous life of their own, that speak for themselves, and reveal themselves in actions that often surprise me—and therefore, hopefully, my audience. The last thing we want is a bunch of cyphers spouting an author's message! So hearing voices, voices which seem to carry their own characters and stories, and writing down what they say—all this is not exactly alien to me. In the context of my everyday working life, I don't see it as especially mystical or magical.

In the autumn of 1996, I was researching *The Southwark Mysteries*, a millennial work exploring a 'Secret History and Vision' of Southwark; my part of south London: the Old Southwark, Borough and Bankside, the oldest part of London, with an unique history going back to Roman times. I was fascinated by the story of the medieval Liberty of the Clink, that stretch of the south riverbank which lay outside the law of the City of London, where for five centuries the Bishop of Winchester had licensed the brothels—'the stews'—under Ordinances signed in 1161 by Thomas Becket (before he was martyred and became *Saint* Thomas).

I knew all that from my research. What I didn't know then was that the 'Winchester Geese', the women who worked in these licensed brothels, were, allegedly, denied Christian burial, that there was an unconsecrated graveyard called Cross Bones used for this purpose and situated only minutes from where I live, and that part of it had recently been dug up during work on the Jubilee Line extension. I didn't know any of this until I retrospectively began researching the poem written on the night of the 23rd November.

Cross Bones turned out to be the key to the work, the transformative mystery at its heart. And it's as a direct result of this work that the site of the old burial ground, which was scheduled to have a tower-block built on what was left of it, is now a garden of remembrance for outcasts.

Nine days before the night of the vision, I'd conducted a group of theatre friends on a walk around my neighbourhood, visiting the sites subsequently featured in *The Southwark Mysteries* poems. The one place we didn't visit was Cross Bones itself, since at the time I didn't even know it existed. Around this time I had a strong intuition: 'John Crow is back'.

Now John Crow had been a kind of shamanistic persona for me since my youthful experiments with mind-altering substances. On my third acid trip, I'd shape-shifted into a crow and taken flight, not only in the vision, but also in the physical world: looking down, I'd seen my friends sitting around our camp-fire in the garden as I circled above them.

I hadn't known what to do with the experience. I was only 17, with no wise old father shaman to guide me, let me sweep his floor, teach me the tricks of the trade. So I went off into the world and lost my way. During a mid-life crisis, when I attempted to re-connect with what I temporarily mistook for 'the real world', I renounced the use of psychedelics.

When I'd first resumed my experiments in the 1990s, it had been with relatively small doses of 'party acid', which had proved decidedly underwhelming. Then a friend gifted me a bottle of very pure liquid acid. I decided to take a much larger dose, and prepared myself to embark on a vision quest.

For this sort of work, I find it useful to draw my own boundaries around which everything can dissolve and shape-shift and rearrange. I like to imagine myself held in divine bondage to The Goose, so I don't harm my body, even when I'm journeying in spirit. The only time I ever hurt myself was when Jesus came to tell me that I could 'not serve two masters'. I told him: 'I serve The Goose'. Then we had a wrestle on my old Tibetan carpet. A word of advice... Don't! Just don't! He's still The Man, for all they've done with him. For months after our wrestling match, my back was completely cricked. But that's another story.

People ask me: 'How do you protect yourself when you're channelling on acid?'. Well, it's best not to get too hung up on protecting yourself because that can actually feed fear, giving power to the very things you're seeking protection from. If you've got your personal amulet, great!—but only if it's working for you, positively, if it's making you strong to walk your path. If you're huddled in a corner clutching it, trying to protect yourself from enemies that are mostly in your own mind, time to throw it away. The trick is to become empty, to cultivate a shining emptiness in which we're free from fear of possession or 'attachments' of alien entities, because there's nothing for anything to attach to.

So that night I chanted the Heart Sutra, that great Buddhist hymn to 'No-thing-ness', to the 'shining emptiness'! Having prepared the ground, I then began writing in my John Crow persona. You see John Crow can go places where a respectable writer like John Constable might fear to tread. I was writing as John Crow, and he was taking me places in my mind when, suddenly, The Goose walked in.

That's the only way I can describe it. It was as if I'd prepared a space for her and then she just wafted in and took possession of it. Danced Her dance. I didn't literally see a ghost walk in, but I felt her enter, felt her presence, heard her voice in my head. She began to tell me her story—in verse.

Now, I'd never deliberately written in verse—a few songs maybe, but my poems never used to rhyme—so I was shocked to find this Goose's narrative unfolding in verses that seemed to slip seamlessly between archaic ballad, vaudeville patter, and rap. I was even more startled to see where the rhymes and rhythms took me in mind. The Goose conjured up the yard of The Tabard Inn, whence Chaucer's Canterbury Pilgrims:

'... went riding for a Vision,
a Vision of Humanity,
Man, God and Beast communing
for one moment in Eternity.

And the healing of the sick,
and the Questioning Divinity
who asks Herself 'What am I
to permit such wanton misery?'

And Compassion for all Souls that dwell
in shadows of mortality
compelling Her to take on very
flesh of that infirmity,

until She's born a crafty whore,
stewed in a Southwark hostelry,
and using all Her wherewithal
to take a Pilgrim's fancy,
and lay with him and play with him,
and open eyes to see
the Goddess that on Judgement Day
shall stand by Man and make his Plea.

And I was in that Miller's Wife,
who pushed her tush at Absalon,
who'd kissed he many a wench's lip,
but ne'er he such a hairy one.

You don't know me yet, dear.
You will, dear, I promise you.
I am a tricksy tart, dear.
My aim is to astonish you.'[5]

That's just a small fragment of what came through, in verse, that night: The Book of The Goose, the first 'Vision Book' of *The Southwark Mysteries*. It shocked me. It was meant to! The Goose is a trickster. And so, it seems, is John Crow. That night I discovered that John Crow was not merely a literary persona, far less a figment of my imagination; he too seemed to have taken on an autonomous energy and will, a mind and life of his own.

The reason why I haven't, until now, highlighted the part played by LSD in this vision is that I didn't want to distract from what seemed to me to be the far more significant intervention of The Goose and John Crow as autonomous agencies. Now you may say that it was my own mind creating these *seemingly* distinct entities—as mentioned earlier, I'd trained it to do just that—but these characters seemed to know things I didn't know, to know each other in ways I didn't understand, and to take me places I didn't even want to go.

The verses themselves self-evidently draw from the many esoteric traditions I'd studied. You could say I'd prepared the ground, created the psychic architecture to receive the vision, but it was *as if* The Goose and John Crow had entered to ensure its transmission beyond my own conscious knowledge and experience—and all of this was happening in this shining emptiness that held the space in which it *could* happen, which The Goose names 'Liberty'.

This is a poetic not a literal truth. Poetry points at the places just beyond words, at the silence we cannot express, but can sometimes fleetingly evoke.

Now people who have visions on acid are mostly regarded by Western culture with suspicion, as borderline psychotics even. And it is important to be discriminating: clearly not everything that occurs to us on acid is a good idea. As with all ideas, we need to test them by their effects on ourselves and others. 'By their fruits shall ye know them.'[6]

And the fruits of this Goose Vision weren't delusory; they were rooted in a lost history, whose rediscovery effected profound—and demonstrable—changes in my south London neighbourhood. Within weeks of transcribing the poem, I discovered that it was rooted in historical truth and local legend. There really was a graveyard called Cross Bones, and I'd been there without knowing it! Around 3am on the night of the vision, I'd been led by The Goose physically through the back-streets of The Borough, to the gates of what looked like an old industrial site, a works depot for London Underground, an unlikely place to find the Sacred in the heart of a city. Yet as I stood there, staring through the bars of the gates, it was as if the bones started singing.

Those songs of The Goose and her outcast dead grew into the poem, then an entire cycle of poems or 'Vision Books'—like William Blake's poetic books, which were themselves inspired by the Books of the Bible: *The Book of The Goose, The Book of The Crow, The Bankside Book of Revelation,* and so on. These in turn grew into a cycle of Mystery Plays, first performed in Shakespeare's Globe and Southwark Cathedral on Easter Sunday 23rd April 2000, and the site-specific performances at Cross Bones.

These verses are a bit like *icaros,* the songs used in ayahuasca ceremonies—little threads leading you through the ritual, each song itself the embodiment of a spirit that works on us whilst the song is sung. I have since practiced in the Brazilian Santo Daime and Umbanda traditions, where this is well understood: that when a song, a *hino,* is sung, then the spirit in that song is present, and teaching happens beyond the literal surface of the words. And of course when you write verse, the verses lead you places where your conscious mind might prefer not to go. If you were thinking logically, you may not want your Goddess to reveal herself as a Whore. But I didn't have the choice. I had to take Her as She came. That in itself was a teaching.

The Southwark Mysteries embodies a journey in verse—so that when I perform the poems, I make the journey again—and when it works, I take you with me. But these verses also contained the instructions, if I could decode them, for what I had to do. And what I had to do, according to The Goose, was to *re-member.*

Remember *Her,* in Her Isis form, Isis the Compassionate Goddess of Sexual Love, and of 're-membering'—because that is precisely what she did to and for the god Osiris when he was dismembered and scattered throughout Egypt. She re-membered him. And this was what The Goose was calling on—the re-membering, the bringing together of all the fragments of a world that was being ripped apart right there in my own back-yard. And it engaged me, far beyond the page and the stage and my work as a writer, as an activist campaigning to protect the burial ground and to create a memorial for the outcast.

Did the magic work? Well, it stopped the euphemistically titled 'redevelopment' of what was then described in a planning application as 'derelict land', and regarded as some of the most valuable real-estate in London.

I'd say The Goose also deserves credit for persuading Mark Rylance, then Director of Shakespeare's Globe, and Colin Slee, then Provost of Southwark Cathedral, to open their doors to her Mysteries. More than this, she revealed herself in mysterious conjunctions and connections, synchronicities, serendipities. Was it just coincidence that every security guard who ever protected Cross Bones, to some degree, 'went native'? The legendary 'Invisible Gardener' was one of a kind. From his watchman's caravan he watched our vigils to honour The Goose and the outcast dead, heard us envisioning her Garden of Remembrance, then went ahead and created our first 'Invisible Garden'.

We held *The Halloween of Cross Bones* every Halloween for 13 successive years. The performance of texts from *The Southwark Mysteries* culminated in a procession to Cross Bones, to commune with the spirits. We tied ribbons to the gates, bearing the names of some of the people buried there, effectively adopting a spirit for the night to then release them with a blessing. (One year, someone said to John Crow: 'Will we get possessed?' 'Er... only by ourselves!' quoth Crow). We do our magic, not furtively, not in fear, but freely and openly, 'lighting the open pathways' for all beings to complete their journeys. In so doing we recognise the innate sanctity of The Human and that if it is allowed to flower, to cultivate compassion and be responsive to community, then it *will* flower and bloom. For what is magic but a creative re-patterning? We choose to highlight certain patterns, connections, intentions, and the world rearranges itself accordingly.

And this is what has happened at Cross Bones. Since June 2004, we've held Vigils on the 23rd of every month 'to honour the Outcast' and to renew the shrine at the gates. Having fought the site-owners, Transport for London, for nigh on twenty years, we started finding there were people on the inside of that organisation who supported our work and said: 'We get what you're doing.' I was recently looking at old photos of all of us all in ecstasy at the gates at the end of one of our vigils—and there among us, was a representative of TfL, grinning away in our midst. We never knew they were there—maybe they'd come, undercover, to spy on us, and then some switch got flipped in their mind. Never underestimate the willingness of people on the inside to help, if you offer them a little bit of magic. They're hungry for the magic.

We hear so much about how London is an atomised city, full of alienated people. Each person comes to Cross Bones for their own private reasons, but what unites us is a sense of connection — with each other, with the past, with the dead, not the history we were taught in school but the story of the Outcast, our people. When we perform *The Halloween of Cross Bones* ritual, we're honouring our spiritual ancestors—the actors, the whores, the outsiders, the trippers, the transgender people, the boys and girls of Bedlam, the mad Toms and mad Mauds. The Goose taught me that they should not be merely pitied—though we have compassion for their suffering—but positively celebrated.

Just as in permaculture, the interesting things, the new ideas and creative energies, manifest on the edges, in the cracks. It's no accident that Shakespeare's theatre wasn't born in Oxbridge, but in a brutal red-light district, Bankside, like a flower on a rubbish-tip. This is our true heritage, and the more we celebrate it, the more these ideas are going to conquer the worlds of fear and greed and illusion, effecting real changes in the fabric of what we call 'reality'.

I'll end with two fragments from the last words of this channelled poem, the original poem that initiated *The Southwark Mysteries*, The Goose's prophesy:

'... Southwark shall arise
naked in Her Liberty
on the South Bank of the Thames
arrayed in all Her finery
with all Her Children
endowed with grace and dignity

the deformed and the deviant
embraced into Her Unity

with Lambeth below Her
Blake's garden in Eternity...

... and harken to that silence what is
brimming with immensity

Unspeakable
shall speak and in One Word
unfold Her Mystery
pronounce the End of Time
and beginning of Eternity

and all Her Children gathered there
in all their multiplicity

with One Voice
shall speak Her Name

And Her Name is Liberty[7]

References:

1. Constable, J. *The Southwark Mysteries*. Oberon Books. 1999.

2. Ibid.

3. Stow, J. *A Survey of London, written in the year 1598*. Stroud, Sutton Publishing. 2005.

4. Constable, J. *The Southwark Mysteries*.

5. Ibid.

6. The Gospel of Matthew 7:16

7. Constable, J. *The Southwark Mysteries*.

Thanks to Oberon Books for permission to
quote from *The Southwark Mysteries* by John Constable

NARRATIVES OF PSYCHEDELIC EXPERIENCES AND THE QUEST FOR 'TRUTH'

'SELF', MEANING AND TRANSFORMATION

LORNA OLIVIA O'DOWD

The insatiable thirst for all that is beyond, and which life reveals,
is the most living proof of our immortality.'—Baudelaire[1]

I began this research in an attempt to consider how anomalous self-experiences resulting from the use of indigenous plant medicine might speak to the human quest for truth, meaning and transformation. But in the precarious territory of so-called non-ordinary states of consciousness, a series of related questions emerged which cut through the framework of that initial inquiry, opening up a space for reflecting on what is meant by the notion of 'self' and how we might account for 'truth'.

Drawing on the narrative of a female interviewee, who took part in a qualitative study about her experiences of drinking ayahuasca, themes of transcendence, a respect for nature and awareness of the interrelationality of life forms surfaced in the analysis. Further problematizing ideas of the 'self' and 'truth' as objects which can be fixed in time and space, the story spoke to the impossibility of giving a coherent account of 'reality', suggesting instead a perpetual movement beyond the boundaries of 'self' into something unknown and unknowable.

THE STORY

32 years old at the time of interviewing, Anna grew up in an Eastern European city within a culture of Jewish and Christian mysticism. Raised by both parents with her younger brother and two older sisters, she said she felt a strong connection to the sacred and divine throughout her childhood. The first thing that struck me about the story of her past was the flow of the narrative, which contrasted with the account of her later transitions into adolescence and adulthood. Shifting fluidly between descriptions of personal visions and revelations, and her social biographical history, the intertwined and inseparable nature of her internal and external worlds as constitutive of each other, was revealed. In Anna's words:

> I remember the tree in our back garden and I was strongly connected with that tree... it welcomed me, and there was nothing dividing us... I was the tree and the tree was me. Except there was no 'I' and no 'me', and in fact there wasn't even a 'tree.' We were just energy, vibration, matter and spirit, light and God... I sought solace from that tree—the garden was 'source.' We went there to be renewed or reborn... all of us... the garden was like a saviour in some ways... I just had a respect for Mother Earth and for our father, the sky. I suppose looking back I could say that tree was my mentor... I still dream about it... I think it was always there... The sense of knowing about what we are and who we are—I think maybe we are all born with it.

Here, Anna's story speaks to the interrelations of temporality, visual memory and the connectivity of the material and the spiritual in human experience. And it comments on the notions of tacit knowledge and the difficulties of transferring or articulating what is known, without knowing why or how it is known. As St Augustine said, 'We know what it is until we are asked to say what it is'. Anna speaks of rebirth and renewal. The 'All' in her narrative speaks to notions of 'wholeness', a totality which, like the garden as 'Source', 'Mother Earth' or 'father, the sky', belongs to a transcendent beyond. The inner experience she is describing is also outside and all around; and somehow comes into being through contact with that which is in excess of language. It is related to personal revelation and illumination, the oceanic experience of ecstasy and prophecy. What we notice here is the wonder and brilliance of a space, a way of knowing, and a sense of being which already existed; as Anna said, perhaps 'we are all born with it.'

Anna's narrative later becomes characterised by ruptures as she describes tensions within her family during her adolescence, when her father left suddenly. Recounting a deep sense of betrayal, she said she felt unable to comfort her grieving mother as she experienced a growing lack of faith in life and trust in the people around her. Her father's departure forced the remaining family into descending financial hardship, and they moved to an over-crowded apartment complex, which she described as the 'ghetto inside a concrete jungle.' The separation from her biological father also signified the loss of her connection to nature, or 'father, the sky' as she struggled to make contact with the wilderness that had nurtured her in early life. After her 19th birthday, she moved away from her mother to study in London. Faced with expensive living costs and language barriers, she dropped out of university and spent five years in precarious states of transition, finding temporary work and accommodation, before moving on quickly. She described this period as:

Intense, eye-opening... but so scary; the people I met, the experiences I had and we shared. It was messy and... edgy... I think you can be too open, you can see too much... there was a lot of darkness. A lot of madness.

Her life story now marked by discontinuities, gaps and fragmentation, the 'upside down' or 'inside out' quality of Anna's early days in London signalled a radical departure from her early life. In discursive terms the story of her childhood might be read as a narrative of innocence and purity, a time when she lived in harmony with nature and felt part of something greater. Throughout history, many theorists have discussed the intelligent power of nature, and the descriptions of Anna's earlier revelations, 'we were just energy, vibration, matter and spirit, light and God', suggested that she had an awareness and understanding that later became tainted by the various fractures that constituted the upheaval of her adolescence and adult life. But without falling prey to the temptation of reading Anna's account in binary oppositional terms as a 'before' and 'after' story of degeneration, it is important to read more deeply into the text to consider what it might tell us about the path she took into discovering indigenous plant medicine.

'MAN IS THE ONLY CREATURE WHO REFUSES TO BE WHAT HE IS.'—CAMUS[2]

There are many places in Anna's narrative that speak to her struggle to make sense of her identity, and rejection of some of the conditions and discourses that produce her subjectivity. In late capitalism, the idea of being or refusing to be what we are demands exploration. As Anna's narrative unfolded, it was symbolised by more shifts as she described having various sexual relationships with men and women, before 'settling down', in her words, with a wealthy man twenty years her senior. They got married and moved to the suburbs, where she said she experienced intense loneliness, meaninglessness and frustration. Isolated by her new husband, who spent most of his time working away from home, she became dependent on psychiatric medication for depression.

Foucault[3, 4] wrote widely about madness and civilisation, critiquing notions of rationality and human agency in the 'Age of Reason.' Following Foucault, Anna's narrative might be interpreted as a further expression of displaced subjectivity. Grappling with alienation, meaninglessness and the apparent limits of her own freedom in an oppressive social-economic system, parallels can be drawn between the picture she constructs and the vision portrayed by Aldous Huxley[5] (1932) in *Brave New World*, when he prophesised a society conditioned by mind control. In this novel, all citizens from birth to death are taught to value consumption and universal employment in order to meet rapacious material demands. A hallucinogenic drug called soma is comprehensively endorsed and consumed by the majority of society, which, as Nicolas Langlitz[6] writes in his book *Neuropsychedelia* 'lulls (people) into a false sense of happiness and imprisons their minds in a gilded cage.' (p.4). Comparing this with Prozac, the antidepressant which dominates medicalised psychiatric practice, we can see how powerfully Huxley's imagined world can, or has, been made manifest today.

The 1990s[6] signalled the decade in which a neurochemical understanding of psychological life became hegemonic, 'flattening out the deep psychological space that had dominated Euro-American conceptions of the mind since the days of Freud.' (p.1). Support for the 'Decade of the Brain' was galvanised by George H.W. Bush, who dedicated the 1990s to the study of neuroscience. But it is precisely this 'flattening out' of 'the deep psychological space' which should be challenged.

Returning to Anna's story, she describes her three years of unhappily married, medicated and domesticated suburban life as 'cloudy.' Operating, as she said, often 'on autopilot' or from a 'robotic' psychic space, she eventually left her wealthy husband, after discovering he had been unfaithful. Describing an ambivalent sense of 'pain and relief', this time bore the marks of the past loss of her father during adolescence in what Freud might have called an example of the compulsion to repeat. She moved into a shared house in London and came into contact with Shamanistic traditions and the culture of indigenous medicine. In an attempt to trace some of the main themes found in her account of these experiences, I will take as a starting point the notion of Endings or Death, before moving in what might appear to be a backward direction to the theme of Awakenings. In the final part I attempt to bring these ideas together under the subheading of Integration, which, I will argue, does not imply an uncomplicated synthesis but rather an oscillating process characterised by contradictions and possible transgressions, whereby subjectivity is reconstituted and new possibilities emerge.

ENDINGS

At the centre of Anna's narrative is the notion of loss, a leaving behind of that which has disappeared as a result of symbolic death. Since the departure of her father, her life becomes constituted by a pattern of displacement and dispossession, in which she is separated from her roots, from nature and in her words, detached from her 'truth.'

> The way I had been living... stole from me. I couldn't live my truth. I was obsessed with trying to be secure. I had no trust in life. I blamed everybody—my past... I felt I was dead inside... It was as though I had a big hole in my soul... I just lived for enjoyment... but I didn't even enjoy what I was doing... I was trapped in my mind and my surroundings... nothing seemed real any more... I couldn't tell what reality was. And most of all I was constantly afraid... fear and paranoia consumed me...

Her first ayahuasca ceremony marked a turning point in her story. Conducted under the guidance of a shaman and in the presence of a small group of others, she said that drinking the indigenous plant medicine opened her up to an intense mystical experience, which she found emancipating and illuminating, as well as painful.

> I saw my life flashing before my eyes... as though I was receiving... messages... from somewhere higher... somewhere beyond the mind... beyond thought... beyond me... It showed me how I'd been living... this force... this vision... whatever it was that was being transmitted to me... I could say a higher intelligence... whatever was inside of me... I wanted to get it out... all the toxins and anger and grief... Somehow the plant was teaching me that they needed to be released... the visions or... understanding came from somewhere outside of me... which also always had been me... part of greater consciousness... it was like something inside of me needed to die... my ego... so that my true self could awaken.

Making trouble for the idea that the 'self' and 'self-experience' can be reduced to rationalist modes of understanding which are put forward by the cognitive behavioural psychology movement, what Anna seems to be describing is a mystery of multidimensionality, a letting go and a 'need' for these illusions of 'self' to die in order for an awakening to something new to occur. This notion of the mystery and vastness inferred by narratives of psychedelic experience confronts us with the limitations of normative ways of categorising and standardising the 'self'. Affirming Ken Kesey's account of the 'surprising and powerful' effects of breaking 'into that forbidden box in the other dimension,' and Ray Manzarek's contention that psychedelic substances 'exist to put you in touch with spirits beyond yourself ... with the creative impulse of the planet'[7] we can theorise connections between stories of hallucinogenic experience and Foucault's project on the Aesthetics of the Self. Rupturing the knowledge-power relations that organise social life and discursively produce the self, this opens a space for the complex interconnectedness of the multiple components that create truth and subjectivity. As Foucault[3] said, 'I'm no prophet. My job is making windows where there were once walls.' Anna's story of her initial encounter with ayahuasca, also known as the 'vine of souls' or 'vine of death' might be interpreted as a breaking down of walls, dismantling constructs about her identity, life and her position in the world.

AWAKENINGS

In a 2005 interview with David Levi-Strauss, Michael Taussig said, 'If you assume, as I do, that reality is really made up, then you are automatically launched into this wild project conflating fiction and non-fiction. The only choice you've got is whether to acknowledge this or not, whether you will exploit the joints and seams, or not, and whether you will allow the sheer act of writing itself to seem a self-conscious activity, drawing attention to the continuous work of make-believe in art no less than in politics and everyday life.'[8]

The relation between psychedelic use and consciousness expansion has been widely documented in medical, scientific and humanities discourse. Studies about psychedelic mysticism and perennial liminality,[9] and psychedelics and religious experience, have prompted researchers to ask whether psychedelics expand the mind by reducing brain activity, and what the possible benefits and risks to mental health might be. Recent developments in research on ayahuasca, including films such as *Aya Awakenings* and the Hollywood production, *While We're Young*, symbolise its widening position in the cultural imaginary. In some ways this mirrors the 1960s' counterculture movement's interest in the vine—evidenced by Carlos Castaneda's *The Teachings of Don Juan*,[10] Burroughs and Ginsberg's *The Yage Letters*,[11] and the work of Terence McKenna.[12] Over a similar time period, we have seen a growth in literature and practices of New Age Spirituality within a Western context. Cotton and Springer's book, *Stories of Oprah: The Oprahfication of American Culture*,[13] and the proliferation of research on such themes as *Higher Realities*,[14] Chmielewski's *Searching for the Higher Self*,[15] and Rose's[16] *Transforming the World* speak to the popular influence of this discourse. And in an age of global digital media and interconnectivity, one does not have to look far before being exposed to New Age practices and healing techniques. The idea that the world and its people are in crisis has led some theorists to draw the conclusion that these times are defined by Trauma Culture.[17, 18, 19] One question which might be raised then is whether the growing interest in ayahuasca and indigenous plant medicine in the West is a response to the apparently developing need for some form of individual and collective healing to address our woundedness.

Whilst it is beyond the limits of this paper to adequately unpack and critically analyse this line of thought, I want to focus on how the category of 'Awakening' figures within this frame of reference. And here, following Foucault's[20] inquiry, 'deep down, what is experience of drugs if not this: to erase limits, to reject divisions, to put away all prohibitions, and then ask oneself the question, what has become of knowledge?' I suggest that Anna's testimony aligns with constructions of awakening in its repudiation of the possible illusions that had constituted her subjectivity and experience of the organised, rationalistic social world previously. The idea of the need to go 'beyond the mind' in order to become aware of its seeming entrapment, suggests an 'awakening' from the dream of rational scientific positivism which has dominated western philosophy and medical practice.

> If emancipation is to remain a project for humanity, if a 'brave new world' is to be avoided, it is essential, Habermas argues, to counter the influence of 'scientism' in philosophy and other spheres of thought. 'Scientism means... that we no longer understand science as one form of possible knowledge, but rather identify knowledge with science.[21](p.45)[22]

Thus it is not a fundamental critique of science per se, but a critique of the dominant position science and rationalism still occupy in our society. It follows then that Anna's narrative, as a singular case study of psychedelic experience and transformation, can open up a space for thinking beyond scientific positivist forms of normativity. Rather it affirms uniqueness, nuances, and complexities, as well as the power of storytelling as a tool for subverting the canon. Anna's construction of her own particular form of 'awakening' can be found in the story she tells about the destruction of the conceptions she had held about her 'self' and knowledge, and the discovery of a far greater mystery. Echoing Socrates' belief that 'the only true wisdom is in knowing that you know nothing', Anna said about the aftermath of her experience, 'the only thing I was left knowing was that everything I thought I had known was open to doubt... And in my uncertainty, I also knew truth.'

INTEGRATION

It is at this point that I want to turn to the question of what it might mean to experience a psychedelic awakening, and how this experience is lived. Pretchel writes, 'We live in a kind of dark age, craftily lit with synthetic light, so that no one can tell how dark it has really gotten.'[23] This, along with literature such as Žižek's[24] *Living in the End Times*, Jean Baudrillard's[25] *Why Hasn't Everything Already Disappeared?*, and Jacques Derrida's[26] *For What Tomorrow*, emphasises some of the real challenges of our times. With some arguing that ayahuasca has 'left' the Amazon jungle in order to show the West what we are doing to nature in the name of capitalist gain, it is important to acknowledge the urbanised Western context in which ayahuasca is now increasingly being used, and ask what this might reveal and indeed how it can undermine the political and economic systems that organise our world. In a culture often represented by destruction, it is easy to succumb to hopelessness. And I want to suggest that the power ayahuasca has to break through boundaries and illusions should not be abused or taken lightly. The values of expanded consciousness, openness and authenticity might be ideals to follow, but questions are raised about the limits of protection and possibilities of emotional safety this cultural environment can actually offer.

It was Shakespeare[27] who said 'one touch of nature makes the whole world kin', (p.74) but the material, political, and psychosocial forces which are currently working against nature, cannot be ignored. Anna's narrative emphasises her personal struggle to reconcile what she has uncovered and what has been revealed to her, suggesting that the ability to live with the unknown involves a constant process of letting go and developing faith. In Rumi's words, 'sell your cleverness and buy bewilderment.'[28] In this way, through a critique of rationalism and repudiation of the fixed categories of scientism, or that which no longer fits, perhaps new subjectivities can emerge.

Criticism of the cultural privileging of scientific values which reinforce essentialising divisions of norms and otherness has been levelled against 'evidence-based' scientific practice by the post-modern movement for years. But ongoing tensions and unanswered questions remain. In a paper on *Discourse Analysis and the critical use of Foucault*,[29] Graham asserts that a central problem is 'how one can remain open to poststructural 'undecidability' without being accused of unsystematised speculation?' (p.4). Drawing towards a conclusion I want to suggest that it is on the issue of 'undecidability' and 'unsystematised speculation' that personal narratives of psychedelic experience and transformation can teach us a lot. For it is precisely the mystery being brought out into the open that I think we need to connect to. In Michael Taussig's[30] words:

> My sense of the bodily unconscious is that it now holds the future of the world in the balance as much as the other way around. We have reached a time in world history when we can choose to press forward with the exploration of this "last frontier," which would like all other explorations probably exploit and destroy it, or leave well alone, as nature lovers such as myself wish for forests and wetlands. (p.32)

References:

1. Baudelaire, C. 'Theophile Gautier' in L'Art Romantique, in Maritain, J., *Approaches to God*. New York: Collier Books. 1962.

2. Camus, A. *The Rebel*. London: Penguin. 1951.

3. Foucault, M. *Discipline and Punish: The Birth of the Prison*. London: Vintage Books. 1975.

4. Foucault, M. *Madness and Civilisation*. London: Vintage Books. 2006.

5. Huxley, A. *A Brave New World*. GB: Chatto & Windus. 1932.

6. Langlitz, N. *Neuropsychedelia: The Revival of Hallucinogen Research since the Decade of the Brain*. Berkeley: University of California Press. 2013.

7. Robson, P. *Forbidden Drugs*. Oxford: Oxford University Press. 1999.

8. Levi Strauss, D. and Taussig, M. 'The Magic of the State: An Interview with Michael Taussig'. *Fictional States*. Issue 18. NY: Immaterial Incorporated. 2005.

9. Shipley, M. *Psychedelic Mysticism: Transforming Consciousness, Religious Experiences and Voluntary Peasants in Postwar America*. Maryland: Lexington Books. 2015.

10. Castaneda, C. *The Teachings of Don Juan: A Yaqui Way of Knowledge*. NY: Washington Square Press. 1985.

11. Burroughs, W.S., Ginsberg, A. *The Yage Letters*. US: City Lights Bookstore. 2001.

12. McKenna, T. *True Hallucinations and the Archaic Revival*. US: Fine Communications. 1998.

13. Cotton and Springer (eds). *Stories of Oprah: The Oprahfication of American Culture*. MS: University Press of Mississippi. 2009.

14. McCabe, D. '"Higher Realities": New Age Spirituality in Ben Okri's The Famished Road'. *Research in African Literatures*. Winter 2005 Vol. 36, No. 4 1–21.

15. Chmielewski, W. 'Review of American Feminism and the Birth of New Age Spirituality: Searching for the Higher Self, 1875–1915 by C. Tumber'. Nova religio. 2004 9(2):109–110.

16. Rose, S. *Transforming the World*. Oxford: Peter Lang. 2005.

17. Kaplan, A.E. *Trauma Culture: The Politics of Terror and Loss in Media and Literature*. New York: Rutgers University Press. 2005.

18. Luckhurst, R. *The Trauma Question*. New York: Routledge. 2008.

19. Seltzer, M. 'Wound Culture: Trauma in the Pathological Public Sphere'. Vol. 80. 3–26. The MIT Press. 1997.

20. Foucault, M. 'The Lost Interview'. URL: http://www.critical-theory.com/watch-the-foucaultinterview-that-was-lost-for-nearly-30-years/. [Accessed March 2015]; 2014.

21. Habermas, J. *Knowledge and Human Interests*. Boston: Beacon Press. 1971.

22. Held, D. *Introduction to Critical Theory: Horkheimer to Habermas*. Berkley: University of California Press. 1980.

23. Prechtel, M. *Secrets of the Talking Jaguar*. New York: Jeremy P. Tarcher/Putnam. 1998.

24. Žižek, S. *Living in the End Times*. London: Verso. 2010.

25. Baudrillard, J. *Why Hasn't Everything Already Disappeared?* Chicago: University of Chicago Press. 2009.

26. Derrida, J. and Roudinesco, E. *For What Tomorrow … A Dialogue*. Series: Cultural Memory in the Present. California: Stanford University Press. 2004.

27. Shakespeare, W. In *Troilus and Cressida*, iii. 3. Bate, J. and Rasmussen, E. (eds). The Modern Library New York. The Royal Shakespeare Company. 2010.

28. Rumi. *Masnavi, Book IV, Story II, translated in Masnavi I Ma'navi : The Spiritual Couplets of Maulána Jalálu-'d-Dín Muhammad Rúmí*. Whinfield, H.E. (trans). 1898.

29. Graham, L. 'Discourse analysis and the critical use of Foucault'. Paper presented at Australian Association for Research in Education. 2005 Annual Conference, Sydney. November 27–December 1; 2005.

30. Taussig, M. 'What Color Is the Sacred?' *Critical Inquiry*. Autumn 2006 Vol. 33, No. 1. 28–51. Chicago: University of Chicago Press. 2006.

BECOMING CONVENTIONAL—

THE LATEST DEVELOPMENTS IN MAPS' RESEARCH

RICK DOBLIN

No matter how much work I do, I will never be able to repay the tremendous benefits I've received from my own psychedelic experiences, and from my participation within the psychedelic community. This essay reflects upon the latest developments with MAPS' research, and the journey to this point. Our aim is to shift the psychotherapy paradigm through psychedelic-assisted psychotherapy. In order to make this change, it is critical to look back and understand our history. We are not looking solely to break conventions, rather that psychedelics and marijuana become conventional. That is the goal we have, something the world and the culture need a great deal.

The Multidisciplinary Association for Psychedelic Studies (MAPS) is a nonprofit organisation focused on developing psychedelics and marijuana into prescription medicine. In essence, MAPS is a non-profit psychedelic and medical marijuana pharmaceutical company. We are using the route of science and medicine to change culture. Our deeper purpose is global spirituality and I think that we have to, from my perspective, find the doors that are open and walk through them while recognising that medicalising psychedelics is only part of the story. Psychedelic therapy does make a fundamental life-saving difference to people with PTSD, to people that are scared of dying. It transforms the lives of autistic adults, people with social anxiety, people struggling with addiction. These are incredible benefits. However, the more profound benefits, from a societal, human species point of view, will be when psychedelics are reintroduced into the mainstream for personal growth and for spirituality.

In 1983, Robert Muller, the Assistant Secretary General of the United Nations, wrote a book called *New Genesis: Shaping a Global Spirituality*. His basic theory was that many of the issues contributing to conflicts between nations have a religious basis. If we can help people from different religions realise that they're just different perceptions of the same spirituality, that realisation will produce global compassion.[1] This global compassion could reduce warfare, reduce conflicts, and build more cooperation. However, psychedelics were not mentioned in his book despite thousands of years of use in spiritual practices, and demonstration in Pahnke's "Good Friday Experiment" that psilocybin can catalyse mystical experiences.[2] I felt that this was a significant omission. I wrote him a letter asking why he didn't mention psychedelics, and if he would help re-introduce psychedelics into science and medicine. I felt like I was on a desert island putting a note in a bottle, throwing into the ocean. He wrote me back saying, "yes, I will help you". Psychedelics can have, through the mystical experience of unity, political implications. That is, for me, beyond psychedelics as medicine; the deeper perspective and purpose of the work that MAPS is doing. Now, how does medicine really relate to this larger issue?

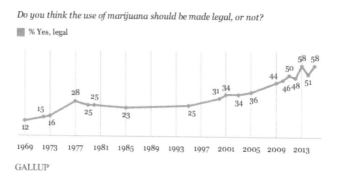

Do you think the use of marijuana should be made legal, or not?

% Yes, legal

GALLUP

According to a Gallup poll,[3] in the last few years the percentage of American voters who support marijuana legalisation surpassed 50% in favour of legalisation. In the early 70s only 12% of voters were in favour of legalising marijuana. The percentage in favor of legalisation more than doubled by 1976, which then plateaus for about 20 years during the "Just Say No" campaign by the Reagans, and a massive expansion of the drug war. 1996 marks the rise of the Medical Marijuana movement, the starting point for the steady increase in support for legalisation, and the time when the first two states, California and Arizona, legalised medical marijuana. I think the medicalisation of psychedelics will change attitudes in a similar way. I anticipate the legalisation of marijuana on a federal level in the US in 2024 and another 20 to 40 years before the legalisation of psychedelics. All that said, when we start talking about medical use it has to be evaluated on the basis of rigorous scientific methodology. I've just created a context, but when we enter the drug development world the science will affect how the regulator is going to react. We are going to try to do what we can in a political context to help the regulators focus on the science.

In 1984 the DEA put out in the federal register a notice of proposed rulemaking to place 3,4-Methylenedioxymethamphetamine (MDMA) into Schedule 1 of the Controlled Substances Act.[4] A group of various scientists, therapists, and others, gathered together to file a petition to have a hearing to preserve the medical use of MDMA. The DEA did not realise that MDMA was a therapeutic drug, and was being used underground. All they knew was ecstasy, they didn't know the codename Adam. Against the ruling of the Administrative Law Judge, who thought MDMA should be classified as Schedule 3,[5] in 1985 the DEA placed MDMA under Schedule 1.[6]

In 2000, *Oprah* had a segment containing misinformation discussing the "holes in the brain" caused by MDMA. The images were graphically manipulated so any area of the brain that had blood flow below a certain level was portrayed as a hole on the SPECT scan.[7] In 2011, Oprah atoned somewhat for the misinformation that she had spread all over the world. An *O Magazine* reporter did a story on MDMA. They even permitted the reporter to take MDMA in an underground therapy setting, and she wrote about how much it helped her. There was only one sentence stating that the MDMA therapy part was illegal, and the report nonchalantly addressed this fact.[8]

Our goal is sales of prescription Good Manufacturing Practices (GMP) MDMA. Our current projection is 2021 for MDMA becoming a prescription medicine. What MAPS is doing is really trying to create a non-profit pharmaceutical company that moves away from being sustained by donations. So, this is my opportunity to remind you that the research that we are doing, for MDMA at least, is not funded by the government and not funded by large foundations. MAPS research is funded by individuals. So if you are motivated or inspired to support MAPS, that's how the research is being done.

MAPS has a rare opportunity among non-profits. We will have a product as a result of our work, prescription MDMA. In order to strike a balance between new drug innovation and generic competition, the FDA and EMA will grant exclusive marketing rights to the sponsor. This period is 5 years in the US and 10 years in Europe. Now, somebody could do their own research for MDMA for PTSD and then they could sell MDMA. Or somebody could do the research for MDMA for any other thing and sell it for that. MAPS' primary goals are to make social change and make psychedelics available as medicine, so we are helping anybody who wants to compete and make MDMA a medicine. All of our protocols are online, our reviews of the literature, we are sharing everything with people. But there is a great possibility that MAPS will be the first one to make MDMA into a medicine. Then we have a choice; do we sell it at cost or slightly above what it costs? What we've found is when using MDMA as an adjunct to therapy, it's really about the therapeutic interaction and it's not so much about the drug. If the therapy costs $4,000–5,000 and the drug costs $100 or $200, the cost of the drug doesn't have a large impact on the affordability of the treatment. The cost of the drug does have a significant impact on the profit that comes back to the sponsor or manufacturer. This model allows for the possibility that MAPS will become able to fund further research out of the proceeds from the drugs we get approved.

Now once that happens we're not talking about a non-profit venture, that's a business and you have to pay taxes. One of the main critiques about the legalisation of marijuana is concern over the industry following in the footsteps of alcohol and tobacco, trying to market these drugs to the heavy user to make the most money. There is a lot of wisdom in that concern when you look at what's happened with alcohol and tobacco. So there is a new twist on capitalism that has been developed in America called the public benefit corporation. Right now, if you have a corporation that's a regular for-profit corporation and you have shareholders, the shareholders can sue the management if the management is not maximising profits. A lot of the time external costs to the environment, to any number of different entities, are payed for by the people who are actually buying the products. This paradigm could lead to a socially harmful situation due to corporations maximising profits. The benefit corporation was created so that a corporation is not required to maximise profits, but can choose to maximise social benefits.

In 2014 we founded MAPS Public Benefit Corporation (MPBC) which will be used to market MDMA once it becomes a prescription medicine. We are purposely not taking investments in the public benefit corporation. Research will continue to be funded by donations to MAPS as a 501(c) 3 non-profit. MAPS will then subsidise the cost for MPBC to conduct the clinical trials. Post-approval, MPBC will market the MDMA, and profits will be returned to MAPS in order to fund further research. This structure is also designed to reassure regulators that if they were to permit MDMA to be a medicine, the marketing will not be conducted by profit maximising entities. There has been a trend with pharmaceutical companies that once they have a drug to treat a niche disease they charge an enormous amount of money. There has been criticism of this model because there is no incentive to try to reduce the price-point because the higher the price, the higher the potential profit from selling the rights to it. The MAPS Public Benefit Corporation is a way to create a self-generating engine of resources for psychedelic and medical marijuana research with a focus on maximising public benefit instead of profit.

I'd like to acknowledge Dave Nichols and the great work that he did in 1985. He made almost 1.5 kilograms of >99% pure MDMA for MAPS' future research, for $4,000. We still have over 900 grams of it left in a safe. As we cannot use the remainder of this supply for Phase 3 Clinical Trials, MAPS has initiated a purchase of 1 kilogram of GMP MDMA for about $400,000. The GMP MDMA that's being made is not going to be any purer or better than this original MDMA. The MDMA made in 1985 is what we still use in our current research, 30 years later and it is still 99.987% pure. MAPS is offering this surplus MDMA to researchers from around the world, for free, to contribute to the expansion of MDMA research. We predict that cost per dose for prescription MDMA will be around $150–200. With this estimation, we project net income of approximately $35 million over 6 years. Which would allow MAPS to become more independent and able to self-fund.

MAPS has completed enrolment and treatment for Phase 2 MDMA-assisted psychotherapy for PTSD studies, and we are currently conducting long-term follow-up visits and preparing the data for submission to the FDA for our End of Phase 2 Meeting, which should take place in fall 2016. We anticipate the Phase 3 Clinical Trials beginning in 2017, and approval of MDMA as a prescription treatment by 2021.

MAPS currently has seven MDMA studies underway, and to date 136 subjects have been treated with MDMA in MAPS-sponsored studies. Four of these ongoing studies are MDMA-assisted psychotherapy for chronic, treatment-resistant Post Traumatic Stress Disorder (PTSD). Two of the PTSD studies are in the United States. One is in Charleston for 24 veterans, firefighters and police officers. The other is in Boulder, 23 subjects, with PTSD from any cause. The two remaining PTSD studies are in Israel with 10 subjects and Canada with 6. Two already completed studies for PTSD took place in Switzerland (14 subjects) and in the US (21). In all, we are going to end up with data from about 136 PTSD study participants to go to the FDA and the EMA and say we think this is a breakthrough for a life-threatening illness, especially people who are treatment resistant. In addition, MAPS is sponsoring studies with MDMA-assisted psychotherapy for social anxiety in autistic adults, and people who have anxiety associated with a life-threatening illness. We also have a protocol, where we have FDA permission to give MDMA-assisted therapy to therapists as part of their training. An important part of training therapists is having them personally experience MDMA-assisted psychotherapy so they have a deeper understanding of the process. We need to train therapists and we can't do it in any legal way with an illegal drug unless it's in a protocol. To me, that was the key approval that demonstrated the FDA's sincerity.

All Severe Related Adverse Events in All MAPS MDMA Studies

Dose	25 - 150 mg MDMA
Subjects	127
Sessions	399
Re-Experiencing Episode	1%
Panic Attack	2%
Depressed Mood	2%
Obsessive Rumination	1%
Anxiety	2%
Headache	1%
Abdominal Cramps/Pain	1%
Restlessness	1%
Musculoskeletal Chest Pain	1%

Data Cut-off: Oct 1, 2015

We've learned many valuable lessons in our Phase 2 Studies. The first and really important point is that safety concerns are minimal. Nobody overeats and dies, nobody has hyponatremia, nobody has too much water, nobody commits suicide, nobody has long lasting panic attacks. These are people who are traumatised and are going through difficult stuff. Several people said, "I don't know why they call this ecstasy". Second, we have very large effect sizes, and several of the studies are over 1.0, this is a breakthrough for people who are treatment-resistant. We've also learned that it doesn't matter what the cause of the PTSD is. We have conducted studies focused on PTSD from a specific cause, for example women survivors of child sexual abuse or adult rape, another study with veterans of war and first responders. Biologically and psychologically, once people get stuck within the process of PTSD it manifests itself as the same disease. Therefore, we will be accepting subjects with chronic, resistant PTSD from any cause for our Phase 3 Clinical Trials. We've learned more about how to navigate the double-blind issue. Initially we thought a low dose of 25–40 mg would be the best approach to maintaining the double-blind. Each subject would be receiving MDMA and a low dose would confuse the participant and the researchers. If we could show a dose-response relationship, that would inform how we would structure the Phase 3 Clinical Trials. The beautiful thing about research is you find out new things. We found that the low dose can have an anti-therapeutic effect, that is that although the people at the low-dose (25–40 mg) level improve, they perform worse than the inactive placebo (0 mg) group. At the 25–40 mg level, people get activated, but they do not experience the fear reduction and psychological safety brought on by higher doses. There is a higher drop-out rate in the low-dose groups and it is not a fair comparison. In discussions with our FDA consultants, we have been advised to compare MDMA to inactive placebo. This is still double-blind methodology, with the emphasis on randomisation and a system of independent raters. Each participant is equally motivated regardless of which group they are randomly assigned to based on the inclusion and exclusion criteria. The independent raters are a team of evaluators who have been randomly assigned to assess the severity of PTSD symptoms via telemedicine. The independent raters are blinded to the placement of assessment within the study, so at any time they could be doing the baseline, outcome, two-month follow-up, or long-term follow-up. Finally, we will be moving forward with a three experimental session model. The first session often gives a sense of hope, and on average we see a larger decrease in PTSD symptoms after the first session, compared to the second. Even so, we have found that people go deeper on the second session than they do on the first session. Some people need more sessions, particularly those who are more traumatised or have a higher level of dissociation.

FDA Proposed Phase 3 Study Design:
MDMA-Assisted Psychotherapy for PTSD

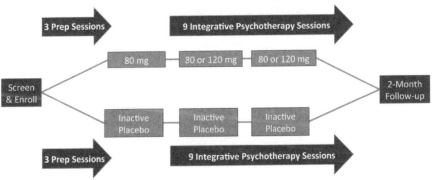

During the sessions we offer an optional supplemental dose, half of the initial dose, 1.5–2.5 hours into the experimental session. As many participants elect to take the supplemental dose and find it helpful, we will move forward with the supplemental dose in Phase 3 Trials. In the Phase 2 dose-response study looking at 25 mg, 30 mg, 40 mg, 75 mg, 100 mg, and 125 mg, the 75 mg group is performing better than the 125 mg group. It may be that at more moderate doses, people are more grounded in their biography and when they recall a memory, they are less distracted by euphoric feelings. So this process of memory reconsolidation may be more effective at mid-range doses. Unlike what other researchers have found (9–11), we have found no correlation between mystical experience and the reduction of PTSD. This further supports the theory of memory re-consolidation as the mechanism for healing with MDMA. For the Phase 3 Trials, participants will be given 80 mg for the first session and then the patient and therapist will have a discussion about whether they wish to keep the dosage the same or increase the dosage to 120 mg.

Mystical Experience Does Not Correlate with Treatment Outcomes

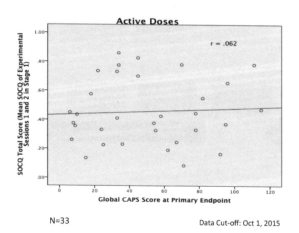

N=33   Data Cut-off: Oct 1, 2015

One important issue I'd like to raise is that we are doing work with the military. One of the reasons is the military has more guns than the police. In a system of prohibition, you look for allies in order to bring in something new. If we can end the War on Drugs, I foresee our relationships with the police fundamentally changing. They would become our allies and we would be able to provide a modality for healing, as law enforcement is a dangerous and oftentimes traumatic career. Senator Jay Rockefeller, who was on the US Senate Committee for Veterans Affairs, has helped us build relationships with the Veterans Administration (VA). We're beginning to collaborate with the VA and we're gaining more support from the military.

With the drug development process, trying to make drugs into medicines, you can only work with diseases and curing illness. One of the best uses of MDMA is couple's therapy, but 'a difficult relationship' is not a disease. There is no way to make MDMA into a medicine for couple's therapy. The first project that the VA recommended we collaborate on is a study looking at a type of couple's therapy called cognitive behavioural conjoint therapy (CBCT).[11] This study is the first of its kind because two people will be given MDMA at the same time, while so far it has only been an individual receiving the therapy. For this study, one of the members of the dyad has PTSD and the other is experiencing problems associated with the psychosocial circumstances related to the PTSD participant's diagnosis. This is significant because the study will have outcome measures assessing communication in relationships and beginning to look at MDMA-assisted couple's therapy.

We're also interested in seeing the results of minimal therapy MDMA studies. Millions of people all over the world are using MDMA in recreational settings, and they end up feeling better. They're indicating the MDMA has helped them, and the question then arises, does everyone need a therapist? Some percentage of people may be able to get better on their own. A study in collaboration with UK researchers will be looking at the MDMA mechanism of action and assessing improvements in PTSD with minimal support.

In addition to MDMA research, MAPS is also investigating medical marijuana for symptoms of PTSD. With marijuana research the politics are blocking the science. If we can unblock the medical research with marijuana, that will protect the work we are doing with psychedelics. For PTSD, marijuana is a palliative treatment which is used every day to reduce symptoms. This is compared to MDMA which is a durable treatment with few sessions. From a pharmaceutical company point of view, marijuana is an ideal drug because you have to take it every day otherwise your symptoms return. In 2014 MAPS was awarded a $2.156 million grant for this study by the State of Colorado. MAPS is also interested in looking at ayahuasca for treating PTSD, and in a sense becoming leading experts on PTSD treatments.

So how do we become conventional? We are training therapists, and working to establish a network of psychedelic-assisted psychotherapy clinics based on the hospice model. We are working to facilitate the incorporation of psychedelic-assisted therapy into standard clinical practice, and expanding the medical contexts for the safe and beneficial use of psychedelics. These psychedelic clinics will eventually allow us to work with family members, and others who are not the designated patients. Eventually I hope that these clinics will be sites of initiation, where you can go and learn about the psychedelic experience, how to use the substances safely, and then be certified to take them on your own. I think that is the long-term path to integrating psychedelics into society. Starting with medicine, and ending with peace.

References:

1. Muller, R. *New Genesis: Shaping a Global Spirituality.* 1982.

2. Pahnke, W. 'Drugs and Mysticism', *The International Journal of Parapsychology.* 1966;VIII (no. 2):295–313.

3. Gallup Inc. In U.S., 58% Back Legal Marijuana Use [Internet]. Gallup.com. [cited 2016 Jun 15]. Available from: http://www.gallup.com/poll/186260/back-legal-marijuana.aspx

4. DEA. Schedules of Controlled Substances Proposed Placement of 3,4-Methylene-dioxymethamphetamine Into Schedule 1of the Controlled Substance Act. Federal Register. July 27 1984 Vol. 49 No. 146:30210.

5. Young, F. Opinion and Recommended Ruling, Findings of Fact, Conclusions of Law and Decision of Administrative Law Judge on Issues Two Through Seven. May 22 1986.

6. DEA. Schedules of Controlled Substances Proposed Placement of 3,4-Methylenedioxymethamphetamine Into Schedule 1 of the Controlled Substance Act; Remand. Federal Register. 22 February 1988 Vol. 53 No. 34:5156–5158.

7. Chang, L., Grob, C.S., Ernst, T., Itti, L., Mishkin, F.S., Jose-Melchor, R., et al. 'Effect of ecstasy [3,4-methylenedioxymethamphetamine (MDMA)] on cerebral blood flow: a co-registered SPECT and MRI study'. *Psychiatry Res.* 28 February 2000 98(1):15–28.

8. Winter, J. 'Can a Single Pill Change Your Life?' [Internet]. Oprah.com. 2011. Available from: http://www.oprah.com/health/PTSD-and-MDMA-Therapy-Medical-Uses-of-Ecstasy

9. Maclean, K.A., Leoutsakos, J-M.S., Johnson, M.W., Griffiths, R.R. 'Factor Analysis of the Mystical Experience Questionnaire: A Study of Experiences Occasioned by the Hallucinogen Psilocybin'. *J Sci Study Relig.* 5 December 2012 51(4):721–37.

10. MacLean, K.A., Johnson, M.W., Griffiths, R.R. 'Mystical experiences occasioned by the hallucinogen psilocybin lead to increases in the personality domain of openness.' *J Psychopharmacol* (Oxford). November 2011 25(11):1453–61.

11. Garcia-Romeu, A., Griffiths, R.R., Johnson, M.W. 'Psilocybin-occasioned mystical experiences in the treatment of tobacco addiction.' *Curr Drug Abuse Rev.* 2014 7(3):157–64.

12. Mithoefer, M., Monson, C., Holland, J. 'A Phase 1/2 Open-Label Treatment Development Study of MDMA-Assisted Cognitive-Behavioral Conjoint Therapy (CBCT) in Dyads in which 1 Member has Chronic Posttraumatic Stress Disorder (PTSD)' [Internet]. MAPS. 2015. Available from: https://s3-us-west-1.amazonaws.com/mapscontent/research-archive/MPVA-1_Protocol_Amend_1_V1_Final_02Dec2015_WEB.pdf

RESEARCH AT THE FRONTIERS OF PROHIBITION: MOVING FORWARDS

AMANDA FEILDING

In the last few years, the landscape has changed beyond recognition in both global drug policy reform and psychedelic science. Society seems to be entering a new, more balanced understanding of psychoactive substances, and their possible role in medicine. Finally, psychedelics are a subject that can be discussed and even researched, and cannabis is slowly moving towards a regulated market in certain parts of the world—most notably the United States. Our long work, chipping away at the rock face of the taboo, seems to be finally breaking through.

However, although there are many promising developments, the extent of the research is still very small, and the obstacles put in its way are immense. These include, but are not limited to: the problems of getting ethical approvals, obtaining the materials, which can cause delays of years and vastly inflate the costs, the problems of storage, and finding funding.

It is an amazing indictment of modern society that these naturally occurring substances, which have played such a vital role in the cultural evolution of *Homo sapiens*, aiding our development of language, spirituality, music, art and medicine, became taboo. They have always been shrouded in mystery, but it is interesting how they became toxic in the mind of society—moving from being known as the food of the gods, the vine of the soul, the sacred leaf, to substances of damnation and criminalisation.

It is a sad reflection on our present society that these compounds that formed the psychoactive essence of the transformational rituals throughout history, from prehistoric caves to the soma drunk by Shiva, the elixir of Eleusis and the brew of the Amazonian jungle, should now be designated by our highest authorities, the United Nations, as a Schedule I substance, i.e. highly dangerous, and with no medical benefit whatsoever. These substances are as tightly controlled as nuclear weapons, with trillions of dollars spent on trying to eradicate them from the face of the earth. Quite obviously an impossible task. So why try, one might well ask?

Interestingly, our latest research at the Beckley/Imperial Research Programme throws new light on this perplexing enigma (Carhart-Harris et al., 2014; Lebedev et al, 2015). Our research shows that under the effect of psychedelics, there are changes in the brain which include the reduction in blood supply to its controlling, repressive network, the so called 'default mode network'—which is a modern, neuroscientific terminology for what Freud called the 'ego'. By reducing its blood supply, its activity is reduced—censorship and tight control diminish, and a more open, primal state of consciousness takes over (Carhart-Harris et al., 2014).

But there are also advantages to the disintegration of tight control—there is more contact and interaction between the different parts of the brain. Different networks, which normally have high integration within themselves, but little communication between each other, start communicating—this explains the dissolving of the normal ego into a state which is looser and less controlled. This state is more conducive to creative thought and problem solving, to the mystical experiences of unification, and to being able to reach and clear out repressed trauma.

By uncovering the mechanisms underlying the actions of these strange compounds, psychedelics that interact so intimately with the human body, we can learn much about why they can be such valuable tools in the healing of many of our most intractable diseases, such as depression and addiction. They interact with our neurotransmitter systems and bring about changes in consciousness, such as unblocking set patterns of negative or self-destructive thought—washing out long-embedded, repressed trauma.

By combining the new art of brain imaging, with psychedelics, which perturb the functioning of the brain and bring about changes in awareness, we have the luxury of being able to know what a person is experiencing subjectively, while correlating this with the changes in blood supply and functional connectivity within the brain. This is an amazing new window of opportunity, similar in importance to the discovery of the telescope or the microscope.

The value of psychedelics is that they bring about states of consciousness different from the everyday. Before their use in research, normal daily consciousness would be compared with sleep or psychosis, or possibly, more recently, meditation. Now, with psychedelics, the field of research has opened up to include a much wider spectrum of conscious states.

A well-directed neuroscientific study can provide invaluable information about how a psychedelic substance changes brain function, and how it may be harnessed to treat disease and enhance health, well-being and creativity.

Brain imaging studies are an ideal complement to clinical trials. They provide new discoveries to drive medical advances, as well as new explanations that give medical research a powerful neuroscientific underpinning.

To backtrack a bit in my personal life, in 1966 I had become passionately interested in the physiological mechanisms underlying altered states of consciousness and the ego. I had met a Dutch scientist of exceptional insight, Bart Huges, who had developed two new hypotheses. One concerns the irrigation of the brain, and the changes in blood supply to the brain underlying altered states of consciousness. The second describes the physiological basis of the 'ego', as a conditioned reflex mechanism based on word recognition, which directs blood to those brain centres most essential for survival, while repressing blood flow to the other parts. This was the first time that a mechanistic explanation of the 'ego' had been given.

It also provided the first explanation of how brain functioning can be altered by such practices as yogic deep breathing and the ingestion of psychoactive substances, to name but two. The underlying theory is that these techniques bring about a change in blood supply to the brain, together with a loosening of the repressive control of the ego-mechanism over consciousness.

With an understanding of these mechanisms, I found I could take control of the changing state of consciousness brought about by LSD—with a moderate dose, together with vitamin C, and glucose to maintain the blood sugar level, I could keep my mental concentration for creative thought and disciplined work. Higher doses would enable more mystical and psychological exploration. The expansion of awareness added a sparkle to my perception, allowing me to think deeper, see further, and feel more sensitively—a whole new world opened up.

I was so inspired by this new knowledge that I decided to devote my life to researching and communicating it. In the enthusiasm of the 1960s, we thought societal change was just around the corner.

This came to an abrupt end when the Establishment panicked, terrified at the new freedoms of the youth. The prison doors of Prohibition slammed shut. Scientific research came to an end, and prisons began to fill up.

The new explanation of the ego, as a conditioned reflex mechanism superimposed over the rest of the brain, could not in those days be tested empirically.

However, with the development of more advanced brain-imaging technologies, and particularly fMRI in the early 1990s, it became possible to observe the changes in blood supply and brain function, correlated with subjective experience, during both normal and altered states of consciousness.

In 1998 I set up the Beckley Foundation with two main aims: firstly, to investigate consciousness and its changing states, and secondly, to reform global drug policy.

I invited some of the world's leading scientists—including Albert Hofmann, Sasha Shulgin, Colin Blakemore, Dave Nutt, Les Iversen, and Dave Nichols among others—to form a Scientific Advisory Board.

I realised that Policy and Science are intimately interrelated and that it was essential to change drug policy in order to move the science forward. Now the positive results from the scientific research will, hopefully, begin in turn to advance the policy. They work in synergy. I also realised the enormous value of the very best science in breaking the taboo on these substances.

I won't spend time detailing 17 years of policy struggles, but after 50 devastating years of prohibition, the cracks in the edifice are beginning to show. When I founded the Beckley Foundation, all 'drugs' were inherently evil, destructive, and antisocial. People who used them were criminals, misfits and unproductive members of society. There was no word for 'use', only 'misuse' or 'abuse'... no acknowledgement or research of their possible benefits.

They are still in Schedule 1, and Theresa May, our Home Secretary, is currently planning a Bill to ban all psychoactive substances, other than those approved by the government.*

As a minimal reform, these substances should be re-designated to Schedule II, to facilitate research and to permit doctors to prescribe them.

However, although changes on the ground are rare, I think the intellectual battle against the War on Drugs has largely been won. In the last few years the balance has changed, the hegemony of the United States has diminished, and Latin America has gained in strength.

Presidents in the region, such as Pérez Molina in Guatemala, Santos in Colombia and Mujica in Uruguay, have called for policy reform.

---

* The Psychoactive Substances Act was brought into effect by the UK Home Office on 26 May 2016. To mark the day, the Beckley Foundation released the chapter on NPS from their forthcoming report 'Roadmaps to Regulation: Cannabis, Psychedelics, MDMA and New Psychoactive Substances,' which outlines how these compounds might be legally regulated instead, to the great benefit of public health.

Even President Obama has endorsed the need to explore alternatives.

Within the citadel of prohibition itself—the United States—over 50% of the population now live in a state which has embraced new approaches to cannabis. Beyond the US, countries such as Guatemala, Colombia, Uruguay, Czech Republic, Portugal, Spain and now Jamaica are exploring a range of alternative policies to regulate cannabis. An additional factor is that the US no longer needs the War on Drugs to enter the countries it wants to... it now has the 'war on terror'.

Reforming Policy has always been my duty. My passion is the science. Surely, the best game in town is to better understand our consciousness, and how to enhance its functioning?

INTERVIEW BETWEEN AMANDA AND MICHAEL POLLAN

What follows is the transcript of an interview between Amanda Feilding and Michael Pollan, American author, journalist, activist and professor of journalism at the UC Berkeley Graduate School of Journalism. The interview took place at the Breaking Convention Conference in London in July 2015.

Michael Pollan: I've been researching psychedelic science around the world and one of the things that struck me is how often I see your fingerprints on it. You know, your name is on papers or in acknowledgements and there's an enormous range to the kind of research that you've been involved with. I wonder whether you could perhaps start by helping us understand: Is there a common theme or denominator here? Is there a central question you're trying to answer?

Amanda Feilding: Yes. My overall interest is consciousness and its importance to the individual, but also to society, but even consciousness has been a taboo subject. Francis Crick said that you couldn't get a grant if consciousness was mentioned in it. But altered states of consciousness are way beyond the taboo. I came across their value in the '60s before they were prohibited and I realised how [psychedelics] can change consciousness in many ways, that we can use them in many, many different areas of life and they have incredibly deep potential benefits.

Michael Pollan: And this grew out of your own experience?

Amanda Feilding: Yes, and most importantly meeting with scientists who described to me the physiological basis, or the hypothesis of the physiological explanation of what underlies the changes, so that one could understand it and try to use it productively in more than one or two ways.

Michael Pollan: One of the things in getting to know you over the past few days, was you describing your past use of LSD and that it's very different from what you usually hear about. Usually, you hear about the LSD trip that it is this overwhelming, devastating experience that doesn't really allow you to be functional in normal life and you've been describing something very different: A way to modulate consciousness and use it while conversing, saving the world, painting, reading. So tell us a little bit about that. It suggests that our understanding of it might be a little bit limited.

Amanda Feilding: Well, taking the kind of basic hypothesis that [LSD] changes the volume of blood in the brain and when you have more capillary volume you are feeding billions more brain cells. Therefore, the natural sugar level that you want to save for concentration can fall and in order to concentrate you need the energy of the sugar pills. You know, cognitive functioning is the late function [in evolutionary terms], it's extravagant and uses a lot of glucose. When we use LSD as a tool to get to the level of consciousness that one could best function at to carry out cognitive tasks and study: reading, thinking, writing, doing things. There's a certain spot where you can get an elevated state of mind but you can keep control of that consciousness. There is a different way of using it, the more basic way, but it also has its immense value and I think that hasn't really come over into society. I think I look upon these psychedelics as tools. I mean obviously a mystic can get that experience within themselves and psychedelic tools are just aids in that way but I think it is very important to know how they work in order to use them optimally.

So my whole work has been trying to investigate how they work and how one can then communicate it. I've been working with one of the leading specialists in the world in cerebral circulation, Professor Moskalenko in Russia, who is way beyond where the West has got to understand how cranial compliance [a measure of dynamic function of the cranial systems, taking into the account the mobility of blood and cerebrospinal fluid] goes down in old age and I think these substances in low dose could be very valuable for the aging process, for creativity and for all sorts of areas. For example, Steve Jobs would have never come up with the idea without it, so many people want their experience with psychedelics to give them a breakthrough and it's happening.

Michael Pollan: Yeah, tell me a little bit about creativity? I mean this is something that hasn't been studied recently as far as I know.

Amanda Feilding: No.

Michael Pollan: And is this an area you are interested in advancing?

Amanda Feilding: Very much.

Michael Pollan: Creativity is a difficult thing to measure.

Amanda Feilding: That's the trouble. I think the present tests of creativity don't test for creativity. It tests an awful lot of things—all sorts of patterns [recognition], tests [of problem solving]. I think we have to really examine how does one test creativity. What I used to do is play the game 'Go', I don't know if anyone knows it, but it's a completely intellectual game and you're dependent on thought. I found I could play a better game, win more games if I was taking the right quantity of LSD and keeping my sugar level normal. My game improved. My creative perception of problem solving on the 'Go' board was enhanced. So I think that's quite a good test if one could set it up as a brain imaging [study], with people who play 'Go'. I advertised and I got hundreds of people who answered and they came from all over the world. At the Beckley/Imperial we're planning to do a LSD and creativity test coming up next, it is among one of many things we will be doing.

Michael Pollan: Using 'Go' or not?

Amanda Feilding: Well, we have to think about that. We have to have something highly acceptable and scientific, but I do think the modern tests need to improve. I did a study with cannabis and creativity and the tests just weren't good enough, really.

Michael Pollan: We only have a few minutes left and I want to turn a little bit to politics. You've been at this for a very long time. Probably as long as anyone in this room, if not longer. You've seen the arc from general tolerance or acceptance, to prohibition, to this renaissance now coming, which must be incredibly gratifying to you to see all this interest in the topic.

In the long game what are you working towards? Are you working towards a medicalisation of psychedelics, or do you see a wider use than that? Is your goal legalisation?

Amanda Feilding: I'd say my goal is regulation. Strict regulation to minimise harms and permit freedoms and that comes in all sorts of different levels. Obviously the first portal to open is to reschedule these substances. It is just a mistake to have them scheduled as they are. Science must be able to research these incredible substances and doctors prescribe them where they think fit and I think that's number one priority. Although medicalisation and the medical aspect is definitely an incredibly important avenue to explore, we have to also remember that around the world millions of people are using these substances and the harms that are coming from them are very little when you look at the scale of harms. We need to give those people the best protection that they can have and having all these people participate in the criminal market is not good for anyone.

Prohibition creates billions of dollars in illegal industry. We all know the harms it does but it also doesn't restrict the use. So somehow one wants to encourage policy change. What I've done with Beckley is try to give policy makers the best scientific evidence base that they can get and at the moment we're doing two reports on how to regulate different substances. It's a very difficult question but I think we have to really look at it with the aim of minimising the harms at every level that the different substances in their various productions. And obviously criminality make them get stronger than ever.

We want to put these substances in the hands of knowledgeable people rather than the criminals, and have licensed outlets with, you know, teams of educated sensible people working the regulations out... like a good parent. How do you manage it? How do you reintegrate these substances into society?

It's a minority group who want to use psychedelics, but instead of making them into criminals, why not make it like in shamanic society? They respected the people who go to the further shores of consciousness. It's not for everyone, those people who do should not be persecuted; neither should those people who want to have therapy with a psychedelic. There should be practiced techniques for psychedelics-assisted treatment, because the evidence is that it does help in many, many cases. Not every case, but many cases, so we would aid the society and the health of the people by permitting it.

Michael Pollan: Well we're out of time. I think we'll leave it there, but please join me in thanking Amanda Feilding.

Part of the talk has been published as an article:

Feilding, A. (2015). 'Psychedelic Research At The Frontiers Of Prohibition: Moving Forwards'. *Journal of Transpersonal Research*, 7 (1), 120–125

PSYCHEDELIC MUSHROOMS: AN ANCIENT WOMEN'S SECRET?

MIKE CROWLEY

GODS

Kṛiṣṇa

It would seem that in different parts of India the same psychedelic mushroom was awarded divine status. In the north-west their mushroom-god was called Śiva, whereas a little further east, in the region around Mathura in Uttar Pradesh, he was called Kṛiṣṇa. Despite their different names and quite separate mythologies, I believe that these two gods represent the same mushroom: *Psilocybe cubensis.* Śiva, for instance, was present at the 'Churning of the Ocean', a pivotal Hindu myth which describes the creation of *soma* (a.k.a. *amṛita*). There are several versions of this myth, but all describe how the ocean-churning process not only created *soma* but also a virulent by-product called *hālāhala.* Śiva elected to drink this poison which caused his throat to turn blue, thus explaining Śiva's by-name of Blue-Throat (Skt. *nilakaṇṭa*). This name, however, is probably a pun on nilakanda, meaning 'blue stem' or 'blue-stalk', a reference to the stems of *P. cubensis,* which turn dark blue when handled.[1]

Kṛiṣṇa is considered an avatar of Viṣṇu and, therefore, a god; but is also said to have been a mortal human, a cowherd, living in a village of cow-boys and dairymaids. Unlike most cowherds, however, his skin was dark blue. The same colour blue, that is, as the mushroom's stem and Śiva's throat. This, together with many other elements of Kṛiṣṇa's mythos, provides evidence that he, like Śiva, is an apotheosis of *P. cubensis.*

The tenth chapter of the *Bhāgavata Purāṇa*, a compilation of legends about the avatars of the god Viṣṇu, is the *locus classicus* of Kṛiṣṇa myths. Many of these are so mystifying and incomprehensible that we must suspect hidden meanings. But once we put on our mushroom tinted spectacles, the meanings become obvious. Consider, for example, this passage about the first time the baby Kṛiṣṇa sat up unaided. His foster-mother, Yaśodā, had placed him beneath a cart for safety but then...

> He kicked up his feet and cried. The cart was struck by the tender, shoot-like feet and overturned.
> *Bhāgavata Purāṇa*, X, vii, 6–7

Is this not reminiscent of the well-known ability of tiny ('baby') mushrooms to overturn rocks and lift paving-stones, simply by pushing with their 'tender shoots' as they grow to their full size ('sitting up')? Of course, this is a feature of all mushrooms but the *purāṇa* provides further clues to the precise species:

> The dairymaids... waved a cow's tail over him... bathed the child in cow's urine and coated him in powdered cow dung. They then wrote protective names on twelve parts of his body with cow dung.
> *Bhāgavata Purāṇa*, X, vi, 19–20

As the *Psilocybe cubensis* mushroom grows on cow dung, could we not say that it, too, had a cow's tail waved over it? Is not this mushroom also 'bathed in cow's urine' and 'coated in powdered cow dung'?[2]

A little later in the legend we find another revealing tale of Kṛiṣṇa's childhood in Gokula:

On one occasion Kṛiṣṇa wished to annoy Indra. Seeing the *gopas* [cowherds] preparing to worship the giver of rain, he dissuaded them from it, and urged them rather to worship the mountain that supplied their cattle with food, and their cattle that yielded them milk. Acting upon this advice, they presented to the mountain Govardhana curds, milk, and flesh. This was merely a device by which Kṛiṣṇa diverted the worship of Indra to himself; for upon the summit of the mountain Kṛiṣṇa appeared, saying, 'I am the mountain' and partook of much food presented by the *gopas*; whilst in his own form as Kṛiṣṇa he ascended the hill along with the cowherds, and worshiped his other self.

Having promised them many blessings, the mountain-Kṛiṣṇa promptly vanished. Indra, greatly incensed at the disregard shown him by Nanda* and others, sent floods to destroy them and their cattle; but Kṛiṣṇa, raising the mountain Govardhana aloft on one hand, held it as an umbrella and thus sheltered his friends from the storm for seven days and nights. Indra then visited Kṛiṣṇa and praised him for what he had done, giving him the name Upendra ('younger brother of Indra'). Also, Indra's wife Indranī entreated Kṛiṣṇa to be a friend of their son Arjuna.[3]

There are several elements of this tale which are worthy of note. Firstly, there are the place-names. The tale is set in Gokula, meaning 'herd of cattle' (Skt., go, 'cow' + *kula*, 'family, tribe'), and the mountain is called Govardhana, 'cattle-galore.' I am sure that I need not remind the reader that *Psilocybe cubensis* mushrooms are most commonly to be found growing on (or, more accurately, through) cattle dung. Giri Govardhana is, incidentally, a real place. For devotees of Kṛiṣṇa, it is considered supremely holy and the ultimate pilgrimage site. Despite being called a mountain it is actually a low hill, but in myth it's the symbolism that counts. Being a low, circular, roughly

---

* Nanda was Kṛiṣṇa's father. His name is reminiscent of Nandi, Śiva's bull, whose name means 'happy one'. As an ordinary word, nanda can mean 'joy, delight, happiness' but it is also a kind of flute, Kṛiṣṇa's instrument.

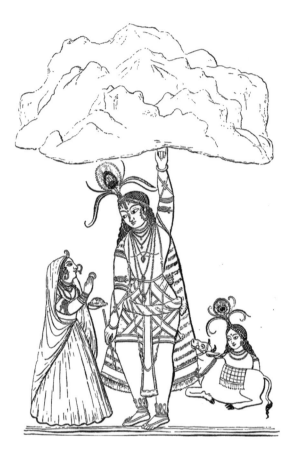

FIGURE 1: 'Kṛiṣṇa becomes a chattra (umbrella/mushroom)'.
19th century drawing, India. (Public domain)

conical hill, Giri Govardhana is approximately the shape of a mushroom cap. So, not only does Kṛiṣṇa function as a *chattra* ('umbrella') by shielding the villagers from the storm, he even adopts the appearance of a *chattra* ('mushroom'). Moreover, with his dark-blue body forming the stem and the golden hill Govardhana as the cap, this is clearly not just any mushroom – he is the blue-stemmed, cattle-dung-loving *Psilocybe cubensis*.

Notice that the offerings which Kṛiṣṇa diverts to himself were originally intended for Indra, also known as *Soma*-Lord (Skt., somapati).

This *soma* (literally, 'juice') was both the divinely intoxicating elixir which conferred immortality on the gods, and the herbal draught consumed by Brahmin priests during their fire sacrifice (Skt., *agni hotra*). The text known as the Ṛig Veda, the Vedic scripture *par excellence*, is a compilation of the chants used in this ceremony, most of which are paeans of praise to this sacramental potion (Skt., *soma-pavamana*) and the plant from which it was made. However, as the later Vedic commentaries (composed c.1000 BCE) provide advice on acceptable substitutes, it is apparent that the plant source of *soma*, whatever it may have been, was becoming vanishingly scarce, probably due to the receding forest. Yet, as the woodland disappeared, new grassy plains, ideal for rearing cattle, were opening up.

This throws new light on the origin of the myth. Given the many indications that *soma* was extracted from the fly agaric mushroom (*Amanita muscaria*),[4] this legendary confrontation between Kṛiṣṇa and Indra appears to document the shift from one psychoactive mushroom to another, played out symbolically by their respective gods. In other words, it records the time when Indra's sacrament, *A. muscaria*, was disappearing whilst being eclipsed by Kṛiṣṇa's *Psilocybe cubensis*. Thus, Indra's condescending recognition of Kṛiṣṇa as his 'younger brother' may be understood as a mythologised record of the Brahmins' acknowledgement of a divine mushroom other than their *soma*. The intended implication of 'younger' is by no means clear, however. The literal meaning would imply that Kṛiṣṇa's cult of *P. cubensis* arose at a later (i.e. post-Vedic) date, perhaps as supplies of the original *soma* dwindled. Alternatively, it could reflect a Brahmanical attitude which considered *P. cubensis* to be 'of lesser importance' than their soma. Then again, it could refer simply to size, *P. cubensis* being very much smaller than *A. muscaria*.

The *Bhāgavata Purāna* tells us the gods' own thoughts in this conflict. Here, Indra gives vent to his displeasure:

Just see how wealth-intoxicated the forest-dwelling cowherds are! They have taken refuge with Kṛiṣṇa, a mortal, and now

they neglect the gods. Abandoning meditative knowledge, they desire to cross over the ocean of material existence through ritualistic so-called sacrifices which are like unstable boats.
Śrīmad Bhāgavata Purāna, X, xxv, 3–4.[5]

It is significant that the *purāna* chooses to characterise the worship of Kṛiṣṇa as a kind of 'intoxication'. Surely, this is the author of this passage giving his audience the literary equivalent of a sly wink. Then there is the matter of 'wealth.' Nowhere in the myth is it suggested that the local cowherds were especially prosperous so why is the phrase 'wealth-intoxicated' (Skt., *śrī mada*) put into Indra's mouth? If the cow-herds were literally intoxicated by 'wealth' one might almost suspect that *śrī*, the Sanskrit word for 'wealth,' might have another meaning. We shall return to the subject of *śrī* later, when we consider the goddess of that name.

Indra also complains of 'ritualistic, so-called sacrifices'. Presumably, these 'so-called sacrifices' were a non-Vedic, demotic, perhaps even indigenous, mode of worship. Note the condescending term 'ritual*istic*'; these were not the 'correct' Vedic rituals dear to Indra. Also, Indra disdainfully points out that the Kṛiṣṇa-oriented worship did not require 'meditative knowledge' in order to 'cross over the ocean of material existence'. In this, Indra sounds uncannily similar to those modern critics of psychedelic spirituality who see it as invalid simply because it seems too easy. The mushroom path does not require 'meditative knowledge.' While Kṛiṣṇa's fungal path may have led his followers to the profoundest realisations, it entailed neither elaborate ritual nor years of gruelling austerities. All that was necessary was to eat the little gods growing out of the cow dung.

Here is Kṛiṣṇa's response to Indra's pompous bluster:

Indra unleashes rain full of hail and mighty winds out of season in order to destroy us because we neglected his offering. Consequently, I will employ suitable counter-measures through my mystic power. I will destroy the ignorance and pride born

of opulence of those who, out of stupidity, think of themselves as lords of the world. The bewilderment caused by thinking of oneself as lord is inappropriate for the demigods, who are endowed with a godly nature. If I break the pride of the impure for their peace of mind it is an appropriate thing to do.
Śrīmad Bhāgavata Purāṇa, X, xxv, 15–16.

It is evident that by the time this *purāna* was written, Indra, king of the heavens, is no longer spoken of as a 'god' (Skt., *deva*) but as an ignorant, proud 'demigod' (Skt., *sura*)* who is also 'impure'. The *purāna* certainly considers him to be far inferior to the likes of Kṛiṣṇa, who administers a timely check to Indra's overweening pride by deflecting the fury of the tempest. He does this by becoming the (dark blue) shaft of an umbrella:

I will lift up this spacious mountain from its stony base, and hold it up, as a large umbrella, over the cow-pens.
Viṣṇu Purāna, V, xi.17

Here I should point out that this legend is recorded in a *purāna*, a compilation of myths and legends written in Sanskrit, the classical Indian language. Curiously, despite its vast vocabulary, Sanskrit had no word for mushroom. Instead one said 'umbrella' (Skt., *chattra; atapatra*) or used a poetic circumlocution such as *ucchilindhra* ('sprouting, wormy [thing]'). Just in case we had missed the whole 'umbrella means mushroom' thing, the *purāna* gives us a hefty nudge in the ribs...

Saying this, [Kṛiṣṇa] lifted up the mountain of Govardhana with one hand and held it effortlessly, as a child holds a mushroom.
Śrīmad Bhāgavata Purāṇa, X, xxv, 19.[6]
In the legend, Indra lavishes praises upon Kṛiṣṇa and then departs,

---

* Although traditional Sanskrit etymology parses asura ('anti-god') as *a-surā*, 'no wine,' the word *sura*, 'a god,' is neither related to *surā* ('wine') nor to *sūra* ('freshly pressed soma juice').

whereupon Surabhī the magical, wish-granting cow takes center-stage.* Speaking on behalf of all cows, she addresses Kṛiṣṇa as 'master of the universe' (Skt., *jagat-pate*), asking him to become 'our Indra' (Skt., *tvaṁ na indro*), lending further support to my contention that this myth records the shift from one species of sacred mushroom to another.

We cannot leave the topic of Kṛiṣṇa without mentioning his great renown as a lover. Whenever he appeared, the cow-girls (Skt., *gopī*) would abandon their husbands and spend the night in the fields with Kṛiṣṇa. An odd feature of this love-making was that each *gopī* believed that Kṛiṣṇa had made love to her alone. If I am correct in deducing that Kṛiṣṇa was a deified form of the *P. cubensis* mushroom, then 'Kṛiṣṇa-sex' may be seen as code for the psychedelic experience. As it is a totally internal, private experience (which provides access to divine realms), each *gopī* had Kṛiṣṇa to herself.

There is an element of the Kṛiṣṇa mythos which is seldom discussed and that is that all of his devotees are female. Why is this? Even today, adherents of the rasik tradition of Kṛiṣṇa-devotion, known as *sakhīs*, are male transvestites. This, it is said, is so that they may imitate Rādhā, Kṛiṣṇa's favourite among his eight (or nine) wives.[†] Not only do they wear women's clothes and jewellery, *sakhīs* affect exaggerated feminine mannerisms and are even considered impure for three days of each month while they are 'menstruating'.[7]

Why do men need to become like Rādhā in order to get closer to this deity?[‡] Was Kṛiṣṇa's mushroom cult originally confined exclusively to women? Is there an ancient, matriarchal component to Indian drug sacraments? This is a theme which has echoes in the tantric cults of the goddess, in the Buddhist *ḍākinī* traditions, and further

---

* This miraculous cow was one of the fourteen precious things created, along with *soma/amṛita*, during the 'churning of the ocean'. Surabhī is unique among cows in that her udders produce *amṛita* rather than milk.

† The legends all agree that Kṛiṣṇa had eight wives. There is a difference of opinion as to whether Rādhā is included in this count.

‡ This is, of course, the orthodox Hindu exegesis; Western sociologists might have a different perspective on the phenomenon.

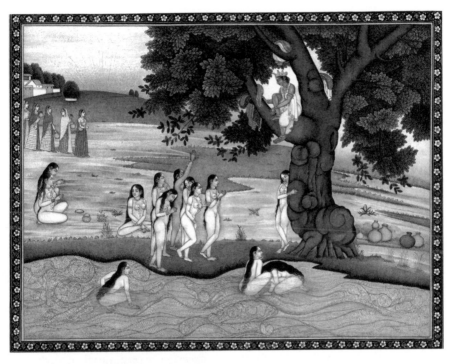

FIGURE 2: Kṛiṣṇa steals the dairymaids' clothes.
Indian painting, 18th century. (Public domain)

afield, in the Greek cult of Dionysus. To make this latter connection, we must first consider one of Kṛiṣṇa's most famous exploits, the theft of the *gopinī*'s clothes.

In the autumn months, the unmarried girls˙ of Vrindhava would worship the goddess Durgā in the hope of finding a good husband. One of the ways they honoured the goddess was by bathing naked in the River Jamuna. It just so happened that, on one such occasion, Kṛiṣṇa happened to be walking by. The girls had left their clothes hanging on a tree so Kṛiṣṇa removed them

---

*   By tradition, the girls are said to have been between the ages of ten and fourteen.

and carried them with him as he climbed high into a nearby *kadamba* tree, from which vantage point he could spy on them. Eventually, he returned their clothes to each girl individually but not until he had seen her naked.[8]

This is a very well-known story which, seemingly, has no drug-related meaning, despite my contention that Kṛiṣṇa was originally a mushroom-god. Initially, I assumed that this was just an irrelevant accretion, an amusing local story, perhaps originally about someone else entirely, which eventually became part of the Kṛiṣṇa mythos. Then I ran across two legends in which much the same story is told, but about other gods.

Birkūar

Just as the *Psilocybe cubensis* mushroom grows on cow dung, there is also a psilocybian mushroom which grows on the excrement of water buffalos. Unlike *P. cubensis*, which, though usually found on cow-pats, may grow on the dung of several species, *Panaeolus cambodginiensis* grows exclusively on buffalo dung. Also, whereas *P. cubensis* is only moderately active, *P. cambodginiensis* is potently so.

This information is sufficient to occasion a reappraisal of such tantric legends as that of the buffalo-herder who excreted *soma*, and the strange abundance of buffalo imagery in Vajrayana Buddhist iconography. Such manifestations strongly suggest oblique references to *P. cambodginiensis*.

The Āhir people of northeastern India are dairy-folk who herd both cattle and water buffalo. They worship a flute-playing cattle god called Birkūar or Birnath. In his essay *A Legendary Hero of the Āhirs*, Subhir Karan states that 'Āhir' is derived from the Sanskrit *ābhira*, 'milk-man'.[9] Similarly, 'Birkūar' may be seen as the Sanskrit *vīrya kumara*, 'powerful youth' or 'young hero', with 'Birnath' being a form of *vīrya natha*—'virile lord'.

Mention of a 'flute-playing cattle god' naturally brings Kṛiṣṇa to mind but, while there are undoubted parallels, Birkūar has many features which are wholly his own. The most striking of these are those which concern water-buffaloes and sex. For example, the Āhir believe that no female buffalo will consent to mate unless Birkūar gives his approval. Then again, Birkūar showed a very un-Kṛiṣṇa-like disdain for feminine charms when he spurned his new bride to spend his wedding-night impregnating his favourite buffalo-cow Parāriā.[11]

Despite this, Birkūar has so many similarities to Kṛiṣṇa that it seems probable that the Āhir have borrowed heavily from the Kṛiṣṇa mythos. Thus, the Āhir claim descent from Nanda, Kṛiṣṇa's father. Furthermore, just as Kṛiṣṇa was born to Devaki yet raised by Yaśodā, one of their songs tells the tale of how Birkūar was born to Yaśoda but raised by Devaki.[12] This legend of mutual role-reversal by the two women does not occur in any orthodox account of Kṛiṣṇa's life. The fact that it is unheard of anywhere beyond the cult of Birkūar suggests that it was invented in order to forge closer ties between Birkūar and the more popular deity, Kṛiṣṇa. However, there are other legends which suggest not so much a borrowing as a common mythic origin.

Possibly the most important tale of Birkūar is one which tells of how he was riding through the forest upon Parāriā when he came across seven dancing witches (Bihari, *dain*) who had discarded their clothes as part of their secret ritual. Just like Kṛiṣṇa, Birkūar stole their clothes and hid in a tree to spy upon their nakedness. When the 'witches' had completed their dance, they went in search of their clothes and found Birkūar had them. The women were given their clothes but they decided to kill Birkūar lest he divulge the secrets of their witchcraft to the other villagers. The leader of the coven did not agree with this plan but then, she *was* his own sister.

The rest of the witches uttered magic spells to make a poisonous snake bite Birkūar, but Parāriā managed to kill it. They then turned their magic on Birkūar's sister, transforming her into a tiger and compelling her to kill her brother. Despite help from Parāriā, Birkūar was mortally wounded. Before dying, Birkūar promised the Āhir people that he would become a tiger-spirit (Bihari, *baghout*) and that, if they made the appropriate offerings, he would protect their livestock. Thus, the Āhir worship the *baghout* called Birkūar every year, immediately

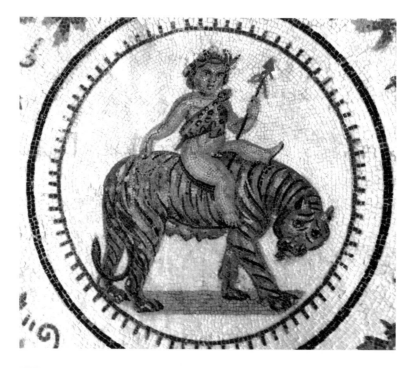

FIGURE 3: The infant Dionysus rides a tigress. Roman mosaic. (Public domain)

following their annual worship of Śrī-Lakṣmī. While this shows obvious similarities to the legend of Kṛiṣṇa's theft of the *gopinī's* clothes, I would like to point out even more pronounced parallels to another myth entirely. This myth is not to be found in any Hindu *pūrana* but, remarkably, in an ancient Greek play. *The Bacchae*[*] by Euripides tells what happens when Pentheus, second king of Thebes, tries to outlaw the worship of Dionysus, god of intoxication.

---

[*] Also known as *The Bacchantes*.

FIGURE 4: Hermes holding the infant Dionysus, whose swaddling clothes are purple, closely resembling the psychoactive ergot fungus Claviceps purpurea. Ancient Greek painting. (Public domain)

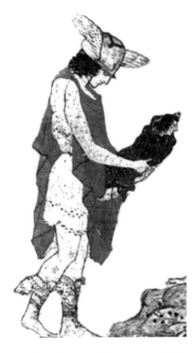

Dionysus

Robert Graves, classicist, novelist and professor of poetry at Oxford, added a significant Foreword to the second edition of his comprehensive survey of classical mythology, *The Greek Myths*. It begins:

> Since revising *The Greek Myths* in 1958, I have had second thoughts about the drunken god Dionysus, about the Centaurs with their contradictory reputation for wisdom and misdemeanour, and about the nature of divine ambrosia and nectar. These subjects are closely related, because the Centaurs worshipped Dionysus, whose wild autumnal feast was called 'the Ambrosia'. I no longer believe that when his Maenads went raging about the countryside, tearing animals or children in pieces and boasted afterwards of travelling to India and back, they had intoxicated themselves solely on wine or ivy-ale.

The evidence, summarised in my *What Food the Centaurs Ate*, suggest that Satyrs (goat-totem tribesmen), Centaurs (horse-totem tribesmen), and their womenfolk, used these brews to wash down mouthfuls of a far stronger drug: namely a raw mushroom, *Amanita muscaria*...[13]

Note Graves' mention of travel to India. Among the various myths of Dionysus, there are several in which India features prominently. He is said to have conquered India and founded great cities there. The name, Dionysus ('god of Nyssa') was traditionally said to derive from Mount Nyssa, on the slopes of which the god spent his childhood. Unfortunately, none of the ancient sources agree on the location of this mountain which was said to exist in various locales from Libya to India. This uncertainty about the god's origin may be connected to the fact that he was a late addition to the twelve Olympian deities.* In addition to his late arrival, Dionysus was also unique among the Olympians in that he was part-mortal.† His father was Zeus, king of the gods, who made a specialty of assuming disguises (a swan, a cute bull, a shower of gold, etc.) in order to seduce/rape mortal women. In the case of Semele, mother of Dionysus, he took the form of a mortal citizen of Thebes. Hera, the wife of Zeus, became suspicious and assumed the appearance of an aged neighbour. When Semele was six months pregnant, this old crone chatted to her about her mysterious lover. Arguing that he could be a monster in disguise, Hera advised Semele that she should insist that unless he would reveal his true form she would no longer sleep with him. When Semele did this, Zeus manifested as a thunderbolt which utterly destroyed her.‡

The god Hermes managed to snatch the unborn child from her

---

* The feasting hall atop Mount Olympus had a maximum capacity of twelve, so when Dionysus was admitted, another deity had to retire to make way for him. (It was the ever-obliging Hestia, goddess of the hearth.)

† Some other Olympians were children of Zeus, but their mothers were titans, not human.

‡ As god of the sky, the thunderbolt was Zeus' specific symbol, just as the *vajra* was for Indra, his direct equivalent in Vedic myth.

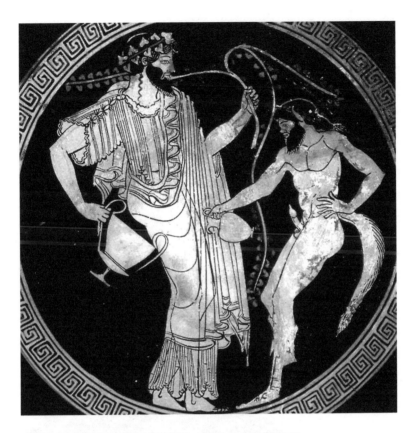

FIGURE 5: The urine of one who has ingested Amanita muscaria is often more psychoactive than the mushroom itself. Here, a satyr collects Dionysus' urine in a wine jug, thus suggesting the use of Amanita muscaria. From a Greek drinking vessel. (Public domain)

womb and hid it from Hera in Zeus' thigh, from whence the infant Dionysus was born three months later. In order to conceal the child from Hera's jealous enmity, he was given to a group of nymphs known as the Hyades (Greek for 'rain makers' or 'piglets')[14] for safety.* The Hyades brought him up as a girl to keep him hidden from Hera.

---

* Note that both meanings of *hyades* have relevance to mushrooms.

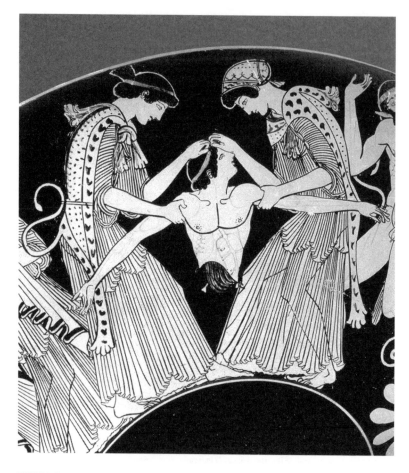

FIGURE 6: The sparagmos (tearing apart) of King Pentheus at the hands of angry
maenads. Ancient Greek vase painting. (British Museum)

Due to this upbringing, he became an effete, effeminate adult.

Euripides' play *The Bacchae* was first performed at the 'ambrosia',
the annual festival of Dionysus, and describes the treatment Dionysus
received at the hands of Pentheus the grandson of Cadmus, founder
and king of Thebes. Cadmus, as Semele's father, was grandfather of
Dionysus. But whereas Cadmus was a devotee, Pentheus was fiercely

opposed to the debauched, effeminate god, despite being his cousin.

The play begins with Dionysus' arrival in Thebes. Pentheus, not recognising him, tries to have him arrested and imprisoned but when it came to tying him up, the king's men discover that, somehow, they have shackled a bull instead. Dionysus tries repeatedly to convince Pentheus of the spiritual value of the Dionysian bacchanal rites,* all to no avail. Pentheus accuses the maenads (literally, 'crazies', female initiates of Dionysus) of seducing men under the pretence of a spiritual activity. Thus, when Dionysus offers to take Pentheus to such a bacchanal, he eagerly accepts thinking that he will witness sexual debauchery. Dionysus then tells Pentheus that, to guarantee his safety, he must go attired as a maenad and they go indoors so that he may don the appropriate skirt, ivy leaves and panther-skin shawl.

This is a pivotal point in the play's plot for here it takes a strange turn. When Pentheus emerges he is not only dressed in women's clothes, he speaks as if under the influence of a powerful psychedelic. They proceed to the wilderness of Mount Cithaeron where the bacchanal is being conducted. Pentheus conceals himself amid pine trees, from which vantage point, he observes the maenads perform their naked rites. Unfortunately, he himself is observed, whereupon the maenads transform themselves into panthers and tear him apart. The leader of this band of maenads happens to be Agave, his own mother. For whatever reason, whether under the influence of a spell or a drug, Agave does not recognise her own son and, thinking him to be a lion, wrenches off his head, impales it upon a pole and carries it back to Thebes in triumph.

It is significant that the actual term used for the act of rending Pentheus apart is *sparagmos*.† The word is also used to describe the alleged habit of maenads tearing apart animals before eating them raw. Graves is of the opinion that these 'animals' were, in fact, mushrooms.

---

* 'Bacchanal'—from the Greek *bacche*, 'howling'. Compare the Vedic god Rudra whose name means 'howler'. Rudra is thought to be another mushroom god, initially an apotheosis of *Amanita muscaria* but later, after assimilation to Śiva, he also represented *P. cubensis*.

† Ancient Greek: σπαραγμός, from σπαράσσω, 'tear, rend, pull to pieces'.

THE THREE LEGENDS COMPARED

Let us now review the spying-on-naked-women myths of Kṛiṣṇa, Birkūar and Pentheus.

One day,
Kṛiṣṇa | Birkūar | Pentheus

wandered
along the river-bank | into the forest | into the wilderness

where he spied a group of women who were naked because they were
maidens | 'witches' | maenads

who were conducting a secret, women-only
Durgā ritual. | witch dance. | bacchanal.

He then
stole | stole | dressed in

their clothes and hid in
a kadamba tree | 'trees' | a pine tree

but was eventually discovered, whereupon the

maidens requested,	witches urged his	maenads turned
and received,	sister to kill him so	into panthers, his
the return of	she turned into a	mother killed him
their clothes.	tiger and did so.	and stuck his head
		on a pole.

As a result,

the maidens	his ghost is	his head is carried
worshiped him.	worshipped.	in triumph.

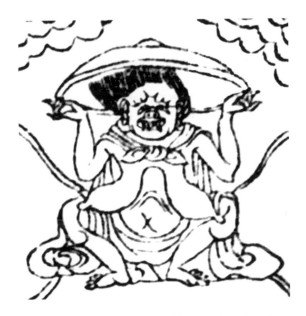

FIGURE 7: A Tibetan depiction of a Ma-mo (Skt., matrika) as a demonic crone with pendulous breasts. Note that the bump on the top of her head-covering resembles the 'umbo' on a Psilocybe mushroom. Tibetan print. (Lokesh Chandra)

There are further parallels which do not feature in this story. For instance, both Kṛiṣṇa and Birkūar play the flute, which is also one of the symbols of Dionysus though he is rarely shown playing it.

GODDESSES

Plants, O ye mothers, I hail ye as goddesses.
—*Yajur Veda, Taittirīya Saṃhitā*, iv.2.6[15]

Śrī -Lakṣmī
Soma originates from Śrī, embodiment of *soma*;
O mother [Śrī], possessor of *soma*, please give me *soma* too.
—*Śrī Suktam* verse 21.ii

We saw earlier that Indra disparaged the villagers of Vrindhava as being intoxicated with '*śrī*'. It will come as no surprise, therefore, to learn that the goddess of this name has a strong connection to the drug *soma*. In addition to being the name of a psychoactive potion, Soma is the name of the god who is both the deified form of that drink and of the moon.* Although, as Lakṣmī she is often said to be the consort of Viṣṇu, she was originally seen as the wife of Soma,[16] with whom she had a son named Dung (Skt., *kārdama*).[17]

This is not her only connection to dung, however. In his book *Hindu Goddesses, Visions of the Divine Feminine in the Hindu Religious Traditions*, David Kinsley states that:

> Villagers, particularly women, are reported to worship Śrī in the form of cow dung on certain occasions, and this form of worship is actually enjoined in the *Nīlamata-pūrana*.[18]

I find this significant for two reasons: firstly that cow dung is the preferred substrate of the *Psilocybe cubensis* mushroom and, secondly, that it is 'mostly women' who perform this dung-worship.

Durgā

The unmarried virgins in Kṛiṣṇa's clothes-stealing episode were bathing naked as part of a secret rite of the goddess Durgā. So, who was this goddess?

Beginning around 500CE, we find the first references to the eight (or ten) 'Little Mothers' (Skt., *matrika*, Tib., *Ma.Mo*). Also, myths and legends of Hindu goddesses were written down for the first time, as in *The Glorification of the Goddess* (Skt., *devī mahātmyam*). In this work we find the story of the goddess Durgā ('inaccessible' or 'invincible'), otherwise known as Māhiśāsuramardinī ('she who crushed the buffalo demon').

We have seen earlier that mention of buffalos could be an oblique reference to *Panaeolus cambodginiensis*, a very potent psilocybin

---

* I have chosen to distinguish the god Soma from the drink of the same name by putting his name in Roman type with an initial capital. No such distinction is made in Sanskrit, however.

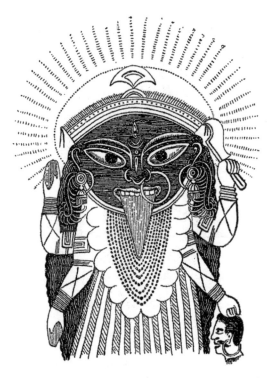

FIGURE 8: Kālī's protruding tongue 'constantly tastes amṛita'.
Detail of a 19th century drawing. (Public domain)

mushroom which grows only on water-buffalo dung. Note that the legend states that although Durgā killed Māhiśāsura (literally 'buffalo-demon') with a trident, her name literally means 'crusher' or 'grinder' of Māhiśāsura. If her myth is indeed an allusion to *P. cambodginiensis*, this could well be a reference to crushing the mushroom as the *soma*-plant is crushed—between two grinding-stones.

Following Durgā's slaying of Māhiśāsura, his buffalo-headed wife, Māhiśāsurī, continued the struggle. Various other *asuras* came to her aid, including a demon called Drop-of-Blood (Skt., *raktabija*) who had the magical super-power that every drop of his blood spilled became

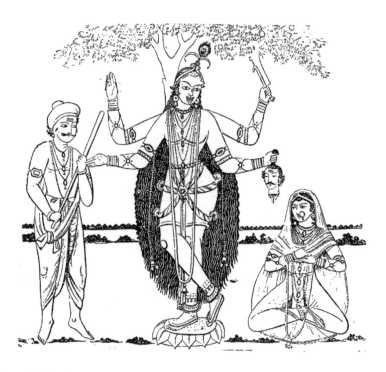

FIGURE 9: Kṛiṣṇa depicted as four-armed Kālī with her hand-held attributes, long hair, and extended tongue. Indian drawing, 19th century. (Public domain)

an exact replica of himself. In order to combat this demon, Durgā manifested as the goddess Kālī ('black-' or 'dark-woman') who lapped up every drop of blood with her amazingly long tongue. 'Blood' is often used as code for *soma/amṛita* and it is also said that Kālī has a long tongue precisely so that she may 'constantly taste *amṛita*'.

Curiously, despite their very different myths, Kṛiṣṇa is occasionally depicted as Kālī (FIGURE 9). Note that his handheld symbols, long hair and extended tongue are identical to those of Kālī (see FIGURE 8).

---

* This is the mythic origin of Kālī.

CONCLUSIONS

Access to the Vedas is forbidden to women, people of the fourth
[i.e. lowest] caste, and the fallen ones.
—*Srimad Bhagavatam*, 1.iv.25

I have come to suspect that the Vedic prohibition on mushrooms and
restricting the knowledge and use of *soma* to initiated Brahmin males
was not strictly observed. In particular, it would appear that, in Indian
society, knowledge and use of psychoactive mushrooms were the
domain of women. In tantric literature it is quite common for a woman
to provide *soma/amṛita* or, at least, the key to discovering it.* Often,
these women are further marginalised by being prostitutes, wine-
sellers or members of out-caste tribes.† These being precisely the sort
of women who, not being bound by Vedic prohibitions on mushrooms,
might be privy to arcane pharmacological secrets.

One might explain the role of women in the context of psychoactive
mushrooms as being the result of the division of labour in ancient hunter-
gatherer societies. As it would have been the women who gathered
mushrooms they would know the properties of individual species. This
is certainly plausible but it does not explain why the sacrament was
not shared with men, as other finds would have been. Did men prefer
wine? Was there a taboo against male use of mushrooms? This area is
sorely in need of further research.

* See, for instance, the biographies of the Tibetan yogin Kyungpo Naljor, the Buddhist
mahāsiddha Āryadeva and the Hindu alchemist Vyāli.

† The Śavari tribe, for instance, were stereotypically associated with drug use. The Buddhist
goddess Śavarī ('the Śavari woman'), is often depicted with a skirt of cannabis leaves.

References:

1. Crowley, M., 2015.

2. See also Heinrich, C., 1995, p.35.

3. Wilkins, W., 2000, p. 207.

4. Wasson, R., 1968; Heinrich, C., 1995; Crowley, M., 2015.

5. Author's translation.

6. Ibid.

7. Hartsuiker, D., p.58.

8. Paraphrase of Wilkins, W., *op cit.*

9. Karan, S., 2004, p.61.

10. Ibid., p.61.

11. Ibid., p.67.

12. Ibid., pp.64–65.

13. Graves, R., 1960, p.9.

14. Ibid., p.395.

15. Griffith, R.T.H., 1899.

16. Kinsley, D., 1988, p.23.

17. Ibid., p.20.

18. Ibid., pp.20–21.

Sources:

Beer, R. *The Encyclopedia of Tibetan Symbols and Motifs. Boston: Shambhala.* 1991.

Crowley, M. 'Umbrellas, Wheels, and Bumps on the Head: A Proposed Solution to the Uṣṇīṣa Mystery'. *Time and Mind.* 2015 Vol. 8, Issue 2.

Graves, R. *The Greek Myths,* 2nd edition [reprinted 1988]. Mt. Kisco, New York: Moyer Bell Limited. 1960.

Griffith, R.T.H. (trans). *The Texts of the White Yajur Veda.* The Internet Sacred Text Archive CD-ROM 8.0, Volume 1, 1899.

Hartsuiker, *D. Sādhus, India's Mystic Holy Men.* Vermont: Inner Traditions. 1993.

Heinrich, C. *Strange Fruit: Alchemy, Religion, and Magical Foods.* New York: Bloomsbury Publishing. 1995.

Karan, S.K. *Thus Flows the Ganges.* New Delhi: Mittal Publications. 2004.

Kinsley, D. *Hindu Goddesses, Visions of the Divine Feminine in the Hindu Religious Traditions.* Berkeley: University of California Press. 1988.

Wasson, R.G. 'Soma: Divine Mushroom of Immortality'. *Ethnomycological Studies No. 1.* The Hague: Mouton and Co. 1968.

Wilkins, W.J. *Hindu Gods and Goddesses* [Facsimile reprint of *Hindu Mythology, Vedic and Puranic,* 1900 edition], Minneola: Dover Publications. 2000.

A SONG OF INSURRECTION AND MADNESS: THE POETRY OF LSD CULTURE

ROBERT DICKINS

Gods dance on their own bodies
New flowers open forgetting Death
Celestial eyes beyond the heartbreak of illusion
I see the gay Creator
Bands rise up in anthem to the worlds
Flags and banners waving in transcendence
One image in the end remains myriad-eyed in Eternity
This is the Work! This is the Knowledge! This is the End of man!
—Allen Ginsberg

Above is the final stanza of Allen Ginsberg's poem *Lysergic Acid* which he wrote in 1959, and is the fruit of his first experience on LSD. It was undertaken at the Palo Alto Mental Research Institute, in California. Here science and poetry embarked on a sublime new chapter in their long-standing relationship.

In the same year the First International Conference on LSD was held in Princeton, NJ, and was chaired by Dr Paul Hoch, a gentleman in cahoots with the secret services in order to study the effects of LSD and other hallucinogens on human behaviour—what we might describe today as the murky psychotomimetic waters through which LSD bubbled during the 1950s; a tool then understood by the establishment to have its usefulness rooted in madness and chemical weaponry.

The best laid plans of mice and men, however, go often askew. For LSD, 1959 was a major turning point, and Ginsberg took a major role in its new trajectory. Hoch and his shady financiers were standing on the cusp of that ephemeral historical marker that we know today as the psychedelic sixties. For all the controlled micro-social experiments that went on in the world at the behest of men in black and white coats, the sixties were about society-at-large, grappling with the psychedelic experience, asking what it could do for them and their society.

Moreover, and of particular concern there, LSD went to work on the minds of poets. Over the course of the sixties their poetry was first imbued with their journeys through LSD's Other space, winding on eventually to become more socially-conscious, providing appraisals of their own cultural spheres and even, in the end, of the madness from which it was partially birthed.

When Allen Ginsberg declared, 'This is the Work! This is the Knowledge! This is the end of Man!' he might also have said this is the end of 1950s Man. He was unwittingly helping to usher in the widespread discombobulation of fixed notions—of personal identity, of cultural identity, and of the identity of society-at-large. A project he soon teamed up with Timothy Leary in order to undertake wholeheartedly.

Before the human ends, however, and before the poet can establish their new vision of the everyday world transformatively back into society, the journey of the experience takes place: as every psychedelic revolution must begin with the insurrection of particular experience. In the widely known context of the late 1950s, it was the psychologists and psychiatrists who held the magic, and thus the ego-defined body came in for the initial battering—the human that ends.

Take, for instance, the beginning of Ginsberg's poem *Mescaline* as a similar example: 'Rotting Ginsberg, I stared in the mirror naked today / I noticed the old skull, I'm getting balder / My pate gleams in the kitchen light under thin hair / Like the skull of some monk in old catacombs lighted by / A guard with flashlight / Followed by a mob of tourists / So there is death.'

The egoic end, however, is also the beginning, and here we will explore the notion that the poetry of LSD is imbued with *transformation*—the end and the beginning—and ultimately how personal transformation through psychedelics allowed poets, and their verse, to be critically aware of themselves, society, and its governing establishment, and thus take an active part in forming psychedelic culture.

In the beginning, however, like Ginsberg, poets struggled and blossomed with their own acidic dissolution in the early sixties. The poet George Andrews was among the first to systematically explore the psychedelic experience poetically, and had a number of his poems included in Timothy Leary's journal *The Psychedelic Review*. A cycle of these poems was published in London by Trigram Press in 1966, and was entitled *Burning Joy*.

The title reflects the pain and toils of his ecstasy, of birthing himself from himself, to discover the greater mysteries with which the poetic imagination grapples. Of his collection he wrote:

This cycle of eight poems traces my trajectory through different phases of the psychedelic drug experience. It contains all I have been able to record of these mental voyages, and was made from the almost illegible scraps of paper found near me on mornings after the lightning struck [...] The human nervous system is a wheel of subtle fire, a pulsating live mandala, an archetypal energy pattern flashing signals through space. So here is what the star inside me said. (Andrews 1966)

The end of man becomes the beginning of something else for Andrews. As he says, this cycle of poems is a 'trajectory', or a journey. Poetry during the early-to-mid-sixties period, whether it be Andrews, or Leary and friends' psychedelic guide books, were very much rooted in the journey as an overcoming of one's fixed identity in order to discover what lay beyond those confines of the mind that are called the everyday and the ego—in many respects, what Joseph Campbell would call the hero's journey.

Indeed, Andrews begins his poem *Amsterdam Reflection* with, 'This LSD is pure hero food / I dissolve into the diamond / The same rainbow that is in each drop of water is now in me'. In leaving everyday perceptions, Andrews finds a poetic, cosmological world within him— where the macrocosm and the microcosm are collapsed in on one another. The rainbow is the meaning and beauty of the cosmological spectrum that one ordinarily views as external in the everyday world as the conditioned ego, and which Andrews finds deep within his psyche.

The *Burning Joy*, Andrews's socially-conditioned ego birthing an identity of vastness that breaks apart his everyday, makes an interesting development when he returns quite poignantly to the metaphor half way through the poem, and says, 'The same rainbow that is in each drop of water is in each of us / Stay on the point of the diamond'. His 'I' becomes an 'us' and he finds himself no longer dissolving, but holding steady on the point of the infinite, the 'diamond'. And at this place, from the point of view of the infinite, he looks back and reflects at the everyday world:

At the peak of its climax the silence is resounding
L'oiseau blanc de mon regard s'envole*
Go clear into that always present clamor
Soldiers, take orders only from the rainbow radiance!
Peace to the world LSD is the only answer to the atom bomb
Bringing transcendental purity into terrestrial form

At the climatic silence, when the white bird tweaks in his eye, there is the command, 'Go clear into that always present clamor', or in other words, the everyday world. The point of the diamond, containing all colours of the rainbow, is the only place, he believes, soldiers should take their commands from. And through LSD illuminating the greater Self, Andrews finds an answer to the atom bomb—that looming, glooming, shadow that was casting long into the 1960s.

* The white bird flies in my eyes

To bring the transcendent down to the terrestrial is where his answer to total, obliterating war could be found.

George Andrews, and the later Psychedelic Left, had found a critique of the everyday deep within the psychedelic experience and it was mystical, yet it could only take form—in this case anti-war, ban the bomb—through their own actions in the everyday world. The hero's journey, in one sense individual and in another universal, would need to be brought to bear upon the middle world; the world of culture, society, and politics.

He finally ends *Amsterdam Reflection* with the lines, 'let the elixir current pass from person to person from nation to nation / until the whole world is united in ecstasy'. Or, let LSD pass from person to person, and let them all ecstatically stand out from themselves, and see the futility of opposition in a unified world. The stage was set for the popularisation of LSD.

From two Americans who travelled to Britain and Europe, it is necessary now to turn to an Englishman who travelled to America.

Thom Gunn was a poet born in Gravesend, in Kent, who after two years of National Service went on to study at Cambridge. Gunn's first collection of poetry, *Fighting Terms,* was published in 1954 and he continued to publish collections semi-regularly throughout his life. After university, he followed his university friend, the American Mike Kitay, to the US, taking up a teaching post at Stanford, before finally settling in San Francisco.

In the US he found fresh importance and verve in his life. He was able to express his homosexuality in ways that were unthinkable in England at the time; he took a new mentor in the shape of the poet Yvonne Winters; and was introduced to writers like William Carlos Williams for the first time. And although he began experimenting with free verse, he never gave up writing the stricter metrical forms with which he had grown up in England. In San Francisco, he was well placed for submersion in the counterculture and psychedelic movements. Later in his life he told an interviewer:

> Everyone was taking acid in 1965, and I decided to give up
> tenure then. I said I wanted to devote my self to my poetry, but
> the real reason was that I wanted to go to concerts in the park
> and take acid [...] I did quite a bit of it with all my friends in the
> next few years. It gave me all sorts of subject matter.
> (Campbell 1999, 38)

Gunn said that he went through a dry writing spell during the early
1960s, and that coming out of this period into more poetic productivity
coincided with doing an 'awful lot' of acid. He said, 'It was wonderful. It
got rid of all your fixed notions, and stirred you up, and you got wonderful
visual images' (Campbell 1999, 38). Gunn's personal transformation
was in part his adventure to a new land, America, and his poetry of the
mid-to-late sixties became the record of that transformation as an artist
as well his journeys to new psychedelic territories.

The collection that included his acid poetry from this period,
and which concerns itself at the very core with transformation or
metamorphosis, was entitled *Moly* and was published in 1971. He later
named it as the favourite of all his works and, poetically, it tends toward
established meter in its construction. Of his collection, Gunn wrote:

> Moly can help us to know our own potential for change: even
> though we are in the power of Circe or of time, we do not have
> to become pigs, we do not have to be unmanned, we are as free
> to make and unmake ourselves as we were at the age of ten.
> (Gunn 1971, ii)

Moly is the mythical plant that was given to Odysseus, in *The
Odyssey*, by the God Hermes—who was disguised as a young man with
the down just showing on his face. It was an apotropaic ward to protect
him from the magic of the witch Circe, who had already turned his
men into pigs. The title poem of the collection, *Moly*, describes the
experience of being bewitched by Circe and going through the pig
transformation.

Years after, when discussing his use of meter during this period, as opposed to free verse, which many of his contemporaries in America employed, Gunn said: 'Later on I realized what I was doing: I was filtering the experiences of the infinite through the grid of the finite.' George Andrews, whose many psychedelic poems ramble on freely for several pages, tried to embrace the infinite in his form; Gunn, however, gave it shape, just as Andrews knew would be needed when he wrote: 'bringing transcendental purity into terrestrial form.' This is, of course, precisely what Gunn did poetically. However, he was also making a larger point with the poem.

To return to the myth, Moly was apotropaic; it was a ward to protect from the nefarious magic of the witch Circe. And, I would argue, in the manner in which Gunn employs the myth, through which he has funnelled the infinite, that Circe's magic is indeed the magic of the everyday from which one needs the occasional protection. The everyday magic, working through the social and familial charms, conjuring the webs and effects of society, goes to work on us from the moment our senses become self-perceived and construct our egos, and the expected manner our identities *should* be posited in the world.

The social effects, to use Gunn's lines, that make us the 'toad that ruts for days on end', 9 till 5; or the 'cringing dribbling dog, man's servile friend' at the beck and call of pre-designed laws and social norms; or the 'cat that prettily pounces on its meat / Tortures it hours, then does not care to eat', killing for reasons other than human necessity; or, post *Animal Farm*, the pig that consumes, capitalistically, everything that it comes across... be it a new television, a sofa, a popular ideal, or merely the story that is fed to us from our social hierarchy; Circe.

'I root and root, and you think that it is greed / It is, but I seek out a plant I need / Direct me gods, whose changes are all holy / To where it flickers deep in grass, the Moly.' As the consuming, capitalistic pigs, as George Orwell and Thom Gunn might have us be, we have a ravenous hunger, which may yet, however, stumble across the *dream*; or, in this case, LSD. It is then we can find our protection and the revelation of who we are outside the magic of the everyday world.

Would we be so lucky as to find the Moly? Gunn certainly did, as in San Francisco in the mid-sixties it was there to be found, and as his poem *Street Song*, from the same collection, nicely illustrates. Notice, in the opening line, how the street dealer takes the form that Hermes took to Odysseus— the young man, near beardless: 'I am too young to grow a beard / But yes man it was me you heard / In dirty denim and dark glasses. / I look through everyone who passes / But ask him clear, I do not plead, / Keys lids acid and speed.' The poem is an ode to the drug dealer at a time in our history when LSD and other psychedelics were openly available if one were to look for them. Gunn gives a verse to various psychoactive substances, but the ones concerning LSD are perhaps the most illuminating:

> Now here, the best I've got to show,
> Made by a righteous cat I know.
> Pure acid—it will scrape your brain,
> And make it something else again.
> Call it heaven, call it hell,
> Join me and see the world I sell.
>
> Join me, and I will take you there,
> Your head will cut out from your hair
> Into whichever self you choose.
> With Midday Mick man you can't lose,
> I'll get you anything you need.
> Keys lids acid and speed.

In one sense, Gunn has developed the leftist critique used by Andrews and Ginsberg, although I think more largely he takes a swipe at a society of both left and right, and indeed of any socio-political manipulation of identity. 'Join me, and I will take you there / your head will cut out from your hair / into whatever self you choose'. While George Andrews was very particular about his criticism of war, and the bomb in particular, Gunn takes aim at the whole hierarchy of social construction. For him, it is a creative and individualistic endeavour.

The power of transformation lies not in an essential new moral hierarchy that is recognised in the throes of the psychedelic experience, but rather as a ward to the nefarious magic of the everyday. LSD is thus a breathing space in which to transform the ways that society-at-large had previously inhibited and Gunn's poetry is very careful, in its form and content, to relay this idea to his readers.

The infinite, for Gunn, is not best described as a point of a diamond, it is unformed space freed of everyday constraints, and when the poet returns and funnels this through poetical form, he is choosing the manner of its manifestation in the everyday world. It is empowering the poet's own magical interference, and the ability to charm the social, just as the social will continue to charm the poet—only the social might be momentarily confounded by 'whatever self you choose'.

For Gunn, LSD had been fully launched upon the social, and expanded rapidly as the 1960s wore on. And with it, the experience had its critique of the everyday developing along with it. LSD culture became entwined with the counterculture and as it morphed into what we call today the Psychedelic Left, it was able to leave the experience itself to an extent, and take the body of poetical criticism. This perhaps found its fullest expression in the London Underground with the English poet Adrian Mitchell, and in particular his poem *Open Day at Porton*.

Adrian Mitchell was a remarkable poet, playwright and journalist, a prominent figure in the British Left, and an important figure in the British Underground poetry scene. He was perhaps the star of the famous International Poetry Incarnation event at the Royal Albert Hall in 1965, which included Ginsberg amongst its participants.

In Mitchell's poem *Loose Leaf Poem*, he tells the reader something of his political persuasion: 'My brain socialist / My heart anarchist / My eyes pacifist / My blood revolutionary' (Mitchell 1971; 97). Political in his outlook, Mitchell was also an important influence on other British Underground poets, and although there is scant record of him being a user of psychedelics, he no doubt would have been in the centre of a scene that employed them regularly.

His poetry was thus never outspoken about drugs generally, or psychedelics specifically; his political and pacifist persuasion meant, however, that he did touch upon the topic when it came to the employment of such substances by the Ministry of Defence. It is here that we arrive full circle in the poetic critique, from where Ginsberg first stated that this 'Is the end of Man!' and the madness of the 1950s.

Porton Down, on Salisbury Plain in Wiltshire, is a military research facility that specialises in chemical warfare and which, during the 1950s and 1960s, conducted a series of experiments employing a range of psychoactive substances. Amongst the tested chemicals was d-Lysergic acid diethylamide (LSD); an hallucinogen, like in the US, largely being investigated as a psychotomimetic and a possible weapon of war, i.e. a field incapacitant.

In the summer of 1969, Porton threw open its doors and held a series of public open days in which the director of the facility, Neville Gadsby, openly discussed their LSD experiments. They even went so far as to publically show the film made of the 1964 Operation Moneybags experiment, which is perhaps one of the most hilarious events ever committed to celluloid—tree hugging by soldiers before it became a popular hippy pastime.

The historian Andy Roberts has noted: 'Though this was widely covered in the media, the story faded away within a week because there was no accompanying editorial outcry against testing chemicals on troops' (Roberts 2012: 59). There was also, however, an Underground poetic reaction to the story: Adrian Mitchell's *Open Day at Porton*. The poem was first read out on John Peel's *Night Ride* show on the 5th of March, 1969, and was later published in Mitchell's collection *Ride the Nightmare* (1971).

The poem is a scathing critique of a militarised establishment that will have seemed to Mitchell, surrounded by the colourful psychedelia of the London Underground, to have been madness personified. One section reads:

We don't really like manufacturing madness
But if we didn't manufacture madness in bottles
We wouldn't know how to deal with bottled madness.

We don't know how to deal with bottled madness.

Now we all really hate manufacturing madness
But if we didn't manufacture madness in bottles
We wouldn't know how to be sane.

Mitchell's repeated use of madness treating madness, of madness teaching madness, of madness attempting to contextualise sanity, is cyclically maddening, and brings to mind the idea that in fact it was the blind leading the high. The media voice of the poem, 'A welder trying to eat his own arm', is taken in conjunction with that of the mad director in not understanding madness and certainly not the effects of LSD. Establishment society, seen through the lens of LSD and poetry, was shown to be a moral failure.

Mitchell must have wondered as he composed the poem: did they realise that LSD had already made people mad? Mad at their leaders? Mad at their drab war insanity? And that in actuality LSD had given those in the counterculture the ability to be protected from the mad magic of the everyday, as Gunn would have it, and that their spectacle had spectacularly fallen apart by 1969.

For poets on LSD, it appears that the psychedelic experience had an inherent drive toward critique which was provided by the effect of standing out from oneself under its influence, just as Ginsberg had unwittingly done 10 years before when he had opened the self-same metaphorical bottle. For Mitchell, the ability to constructively step out was what the officers and scientists at Porton Down had failed to recognise, but which had filtered out into popular society, and had become an ironic and humorous anger in light of their bottled madness.

If, of course, you can choose to be whatever self you want to be— left, right, or simply high—then being able to constructively critique one's self, one's poetry, one's society, is as far from madness as one might find. The trippers and the poets had learnt a lesson, which they believed those in power had not, and as a nugget of knowledge this is perhaps best summed up by Roger McGough's *Poem for National LSD Week*: 'Mind, how you go.'

Sources:

Andrews, George. *Burning Joy*. London. Tigram Press. 1966.

Campbell, James. *Thom Gunn in conversation with James Campbell*. Between the Lines. 1999.

Ginsberg, Allen. *Collected Poems* 1947–1997. London. Harper Perennial Modern Classics. 2007.

Gunn, Thom. *Moly*. London. Faber and Faber. 1971.

Gunn, Thom. Thom Gunn on Moly. *Poetry Book Society:* http://www.poetrybooks.co.uk/poetry_portal/from_the_archives_thom_gunn_on_moly_1971 [Accessed 6.1.2016] 1971ii

Lee, Martin A and Bruce Shlain. *Acid Dreams: The complete social history of LSD*. New York. Grove Press. 1985.

Mitchell, Adrian. *Ride the Nightmare*. London. Jonathan Cape. 1971.

Roberts, Andy. Albion Dreaming: *A popular history of LSD in Britain*. Marshall Cavendish. 2012.

THE REAL SECRET OF MAGIC:

WILLIAM BURROUGHS, TERENCE MCKENNA, AND THE SYNTACTICAL NATURE OF REALITY

LUKE GOAMAN-DODSON

Thank you to my fellow panellists today, it's been a really rejuvenating meander through various pathways of the counterculture on what I call the comedown slot of 10:30 on a Sunday morning, and particularly to Roger [Keen] for his talk, which so beautifully elucidated the connection between the Beats and the psychedelic movement. My talk will be a kind of zooming in and branching out from one particular facet of that relationship, in terms of the relationship between William Burroughs and Terence McKenna, and this theme of the 'syntactical nature of reality', so that reality is essentially a linguistic construct. Something I want to tease out from this is that Burroughs and McKenna were, on one level, trying to escape from words and language, but in a complicated way and I'm going to problematize that.

So, you've got Burroughs as this kind of elder statesman of the Beat movement, who helped to open up this cultural pathway into the Amazon, for better or worse, with *The Yage Letters*, and in his experiments with yage he had these visions, some of which went into certain sections of *Naked Lunch*. What he saw was this city called the Composite City of Interzone, and he describes it as a 'place where the unknown past and the emergent future meet in a vibrating soundless hum' (1993: 91), where Mongol yurts and South Pacific huts house 'bureaucrats of spectral departments, officials of unconstituted police states, a Lesbian dwarf who has perfected operation Bangutot, the lung erection that strangles a sleeping enemy' and 'black marketeers of World War 3' (93). So you have this attractively repellent collision of the past and the future that's mirrored in McKenna's concept of the archaic revival, this idea that as we head into the impossibly bizarre future that is the 13th bak'tun of the Mayan calendar, we're going back to our ancestral past and reviving these kinds of tradition.

So to go back to the syntactical nature of reality; that term comes from this quote by McKenna, where he says, 'what the alien voice in the psychedelic experience wants to reveal is the syntactical nature of reality. That the real secret of magic, is that the world is made of words, and that if you know the words that the world is made of, you make of it, whatever you wish!' (McKenna 1993).

This was in the context of a DMT trip, in which McKenna encountered what he described as linguistic constructs solidified, these dribbling basketball Faberge egg machine elves, and they taught him how to manifest objects in this space through sound, through language, through communication, so that the sounds that he uttered, and he did this kind of glossolalia when he was talking about it, became physical objects.

So we're beyond semiotics here, and into the realm of words that signify themselves, that are objects in themselves, and reflecting on his experience McKenna came to the conclusion that meaning and language are two separate things, and this brings us to the cut-up technique. Now the cut-up technique was developed by the Dadaists originally, in the early 20th century, and it was a way of separating language from comprehensible meaning, to just divorce words from any understanding, any kind of signification. Brion Gysin stumbled upon this procedure accidentally, and him and Burroughs developed it as a magical procedure or technique of cutting through reality by cutting through words or film, any kind of text. Burroughs wrote to a friend 'I tell you, boss, you write it and it happens' (Morgan 1992: 323), and did these experiments, [for example, one] where he would launch an attack on a café for serving 'abominable cheesecake' and he launched an attack and did filming and recording of this café, and he spliced it up with riots and war footage and stuff like that, and the café eventually closed. (321) He did the same thing to the Scientology office, he was actually involved in Scientology to a certain extent, but then he decided it was another load of control system bullshit, so he launched an attack on the Scientology building, and he was this weird Beat guy hanging out with his camera, and doing all this stuff, and the Scientology office had to move from where it was to where it is now (ibid.); I can't exactly remember where that is, because I haven't had my thetans checked in a little while.

But it goes even deeper than this because for Burroughs the word represents control and limitation and spiritual bondage almost, because Burroughs was a sort of self-confessed Gnostic, or Manichean; at one point in his life he described himself as a Gnostic, and he had this very dualistic understanding of reality. So he was always trying to sort of disrupt these control systems, and trying to stabilise, to achieve mental silence. He spoke about how difficult it was to get to this proper state of quietude inside your own mind, your own being; so came this exhortation to 'rub out the word', and much of these ideas come from a chap called Alfred Korzybski, who was a Polish-American theorist, who developed this theory of General Semantics, which is different from semantics. It's a sort of mish-mash of semantic theory and self-help technique, of trying to change your own nature by changing the language that you use in relationship to your reality so you're changing your reality effectively. He coined the phrase 'the map is not the territory', and Burroughs attended his seminars, and took a lot from Korzybski in this process. And I should also point out that Burroughs' uncle Ivy Lee was a spin doctor who is regarded by some as the father of modern public relations and he actually had links to the Third Reich, and companies that were making Zyklon B and all of this kind of shit, and this puts a bit of context onto Burroughs' very dark view of control, language, and manipulation. Something I want to give you a sense of is this sort of palette of colours where McKenna cuts this very golden, innocent, gnomish figure, and then Burroughs in his fedora, and his black shirt, you've got this different palette, which is shown in their musical collaborations. You've got McKenna recording with the Shamen, and Zuvuya, and sort of acid house and ambient, and then you've got Burroughs recording with industrial-rockers like Ministry and Kurt Cobain, and hip-hop like Disposable Heroes of Hiphoprisy.

The cut-up is more than a way of divining the future or disrupting the lives of London café owners or Scientologists, it's a way of slicing through the constricting patterns that impede us politically, socially, psychologically, mystically, and it reaches a zenith in Burroughs's *Nova* trilogy, the cut-up trilogy, where he takes the literary techniques he's using, and he transfers them into the story, so they become part of the story. They become means of doing stuff in the stories, which are these Manichean struggles between the forces of liberation and forces of oppression. There's one particular chapter I want to read from, from *The Soft Machine*, called 'The Mayan Caper', where cut-ups are portrayed as a means of linguistic time-travel, so he cuts himself up with another person through recording and stuff, and then eventually they become one body, and then he goes back in time to the heyday of the Mayan priesthood, the Mayan civilisation. The calendar forms this linguistic control system and he uses the cut-up technique to start this revolution and he writes like this:

'Cut word lines-Cut music lines-Smash the control images-Smash the control machines-Burn the books-Kill the priests-Kill!-Kill!-Kill!'

Inexorably as the machine had controlled thought feeling and sensory impressions of the workers, the machine now gave the order to dismantle itself and kill the priests—I had the satisfaction of seeing the overseer pegged out in the field, his intestines perforated with hot planting sticks and crammed with corn—I broke out my camera gun and rushed the temple—This weapon takes and vibrates image to radiostatic—You see the priests were nothing but word and image, an old film rolling on and on with dead actors—Priests and temple guards went up in silver smoke as I blasted my way into the control room and burned the codices—Earthquake tremors under my feet I got out of there fast, blocks of limestone raining all around me— A great weight fell from the sky, winds of the earth whipping palm trees to the ground—Tidal waves rolled over the Mayan control calendar. (1995: 57)

So you've got these ideas of the Mayan calendar as this total control system; he was fascinated by this thing that everything that you did on a certain day was predetermined by the calendar, so he created the Mayan priesthood into his own science-fiction projection of everything he thought was bad in these systems of control, and they have these punishments where they put people in ovens, harking back to Nazi atrocities, and 'Death By Centipede' as well, he had this thing about centipedes, he really didn't like them...

But all of this, with the Mayan calendar and the apocalypse and everything is starting to ring some bells when it comes to McKenna, for anyone who has read McKenna or has listened to his interestingly staccato way of speaking. McKenna generally has a more positive view of Mayan civilisation than Burroughs, and a more positive view of a lot of things than Burroughs... It is interesting that Burroughs anticipated the cultural importance of the Mayan calendar, many decades before the 2012 thing came up, mostly through McKenna and his 'Timewave Zero'. So compare Burroughs's Mayan apocalypse to McKenna's answer when queried about his 2012 predictions. So he says:

'If you *really* understand what I'm saying, you would understand it can't be said. It's a prediction of an unpredictable event.' The event will be 'some enormously reality-rearranging thing.' Scientists will invent a truly intelligent computer, or a time-travel machine. Perhaps we will be visited by an alien spaceship, or an asteroid. 'I don't know if it's built into the laws of spacetime, or it's generated out of human inventiveness, or whether it's a mile and a half wide and arrives unexpectedly in the center of North America.' (Horgan 2012)

McKenna's a bit of a tricky one to pin down in many ways, as Ralph Abraham and Rupert Sheldrake found out in those trialogues. [McKenna's] theories about 'Habit' and 'Novelty' led him to assign 'Habit' the status of 'Bad' and 'Novelty' the status of 'Good', so with any spike in 'Novelty' he would see that as being good even if it was some huge apocalyptic alien interdimensional space war or something.

For McKenna the apocalypse might not necessarily be all that bad, as for Burroughs. It's also worth mentioning that both Burroughs and McKenna felt that some kind of technological singularity might be desirable, or maybe inevitable to some degree. Both were really influential in this kind of 'Cyberia', cyberdelia movement of the 80s and 90s, segueing with Gemma [Farrell's] talk about the history of British psytrance, and McKenna was a huge figure in this... and Burroughs as well, and you had magazines like *High Frontiers* and *Mondo 2000*, and Timothy Leary's pronouncements that computers were going to be the new LSD. So McKenna in what as far as my current research has led me to believe, and this could be corrected, but as far as I can tell, the only direct contact, or rather indirect contact, that McKenna had with Burroughs was [a set of] questions that McKenna, along with R.U. Sirius, *Mondo 2000* founder, answered for a late 80s interview published in *High Frontiers*, in response to the question *What do you think is the direction of mind technologies in terms of drugs and surgical implants, external technologies and techniques?* Burroughs replied, 'There is no limit to control of thought, feeling and apparent sensory perceptions.' (Bray 1987)

And with a follow-up question regarding whether these technologies could help humanity get to a higher level of functioning, Burroughs responded that 'humanity is a meaningless abstraction. Are you talking about Columbians in an earthquake, Ethiopians in a famine, Americans in a country club, ethnic minorities in a ghetto? The punctuationalist theory of evolution seems to point to the fact that changes occur in small isolated groups and the tendency is towards standardization'. (ibid.) So Burroughs was kind of evading this millenarianism... saying that, you know, it's too complex to say that these technologies are innately one thing or the other, they have different manifestations in different areas with different people at different times.

So you've got Burroughs and McKenna taken up as senior figures in this sort of 'psychedelic cyberpunk' counter culture, which starts to emerge in the 80s and 90s, with acid house and rave and chaos magick and these sorts of things, and Burroughs's ideas of magick are echoed in chaos magick as well. Burroughs is more cautious and elusive about [technological singularity] than McKenna who predicted that we were hurtling towards a period of unprecedented evolution, and he says in *The Archaic Revival*:

The two concepts, drugs and computers, are migrating toward each other. If you add in the concept 'person' and say these three concepts—drugs, computer, and person—are migrating toward each other, then you realize that the monkey body is still holding a lot of our linguistic structure in place. (1991: 19)

And as a metaphor for how this post-singularity human might communicate, he uses the octopus, because the octopus changes colour as a means of communicating, and he continues:

A richer notion of telepathy would be if you could see my words, rather than hear them—if they were actually sculptural objects. I would make an utterance, then you and I would stand and regard this utterance from all angles. There would be no ambiguity. And this is exactly what is going on with the octopi. (22)

I don't know how the octopi would feel about that, their communication might have all kinds of misinterpretations, especially if they're married or whatever. But it's interesting to compare also that in the latter part of his life Burroughs became interested in Egyptology, which he explored in *The Western Lands*, and he was particularly engaged with this idea of the hieroglyph as this pictorial method of communication. And by the way, if this talk seems a bit rambly, and ad hoc, and incoherent, just imagine I'm using the cut-up technique, and then it's alright; you can get away with anything, it's brilliant.

So you've got these ideas about language shaping our perceptions of reality, it's all paralleled to some extent by these developments in post-modern theories, and post-structuralism, and Foucault's ideas of 'discourses of power', Lacan saying the unconscious is structured like a language, Derrida's deconstruction, and things like this. Another interesting parallel that I find is the rise of the neo-Luddite, or green anarchist, anarcho-primitivist movement, which is the direct anti-thesis of the techno-utopian, transhumanist, cyberdelic type philosophy, and says no, we're going in the wrong direction, we need less technology, we need to smash the machines, as Burroughs said, get rid of them, and go back to the Stone Age. One of the leading proponents of this philosophy, American anarchist writer John Zerzan, even goes to the extent as to suggest that language and symbolic thought might have to be erased in order to achieve a truly egalitarian society, which ties in with this sense of escaping the word, escaping language. And it's also interesting that McKenna spoke about history coming to an end in the early 90s when Francis Fukuyama declares it's the end of history, with the difference being that Francis Fukuyama was talking about the spread of liberal capitalism, and not a massive rush of endogenous DMT that would send everyone off in the same endlessly transforming hyperspace, which is a bit different.

So I want to finish off by coming back to this sense of trying to escape the word, because there's a moment in James Joyce's *Ulysses* where Stephen Dedalus says 'History is a nightmare from which I am trying to escape',* very evocative statement, and just from my own reading, there is a degree to which McKenna and Burroughs were

---

* Correction: the actual quote is 'History is a nightmare from which I am trying to *awake*'.

striving to transcend history, and culture and language and things like that, but in a complicated way. McKenna looked to a future where communication could be transformed through telepathy, when the nightmare of history would end in 2012, not sure if it's happened yet but you know, time will tell, and we could break free from the virtual reality of culture, he said in his conversation with Ram Dass, he said 'Culture is a virtual reality made of language' (McKenna 1993 (2)). But as I say, it's complicated, they were both writers and they dealt with words, so they were ambivalent about it. Burroughs turned down an offer to go on a Buddhist retreat with Chögyam Trungpa when he found out he wouldn't be able to take any notebooks or anything like that. He said he would prefer to be a writer than to be enlightened which is... fair enough... and it's also interesting that Bruce Damer considered the zenith of McKenna's career to be the wordless kind of overtone singing that he did with Lost At Last in the late 90s,[†] that he'd finally transcended all the words and concepts and philosophies and had gone to this direct level, and this ties in with Colin Turnbull's observation that the highest songs of the Congolese pygmies are the ones that don't have words, this immediate, direct communication.

So I think, at this point, where we've gone from a discussion of language to the wordless point, it's probably about time for me to wrap it up, so thank you!

---

† During a spoken word segment of these performances, McKenna mentions Uranian Willy, a character from Burroughs's *Nova* trilogy.

References:

Burroughs, W.S. *Naked Lunch*. London: Flamingo. 1993.

Burroughs, W.S. *The Soft Machine*. London: Flamingo. 1995.

Bray, F. 'William S. Burroughs in High Frontiers 1987 about Mind Technologies'. 1987. Accessed from: tinyurl.com/hs4ogaw

Horgan, J. 'Timewave Zero: Did Terence McKenna really believe in all that 2012 prophecy stuff?'. 2012. Accessed from tinyurl.com/cyyyfuy

McKenna, T. *The Archaic Revival*. San Francisco: HarperCollins. 1991.

McKenna, T. 'Alien Dreamtime'. Live recording. 1993.

McKenna, T. 'Terence McKenna—Prague Gnosis'. Live recording. 1993.

Morgan, T. *Literary Outlaw: The Life and Times of William S. Burroughs*. London: Pimlico. 1992.

Sources:

Burroughs, W.S. *Nova Express*. London: Penguin. 2010.

Burroughs, W.S. *The Ticket that Exploded*. New York: Grove. 1987.

Burroughs, W.S. and Ginsberg, A. *The Yage Letters*. San Francisco: City Lights. 1975.

Burroughs, W.S., Gysin, B. *The Third Mind*. New York: Viking. 1978.

Burroughs, W.S. *Word Virus: The William Burroughs Reader*. Grauerholz, J., Silverberg, I. (eds). London: Flamingo.

Keen, R. 'The Soundless Hum: Psychonautic Underpinnings of William Burroughs's Naked Lunch'. *PsyPress UK*. 2013 Vol. 2.

Keen, R. 'Beats on Acid'. *PsyPress UK*. 2014 Vol. 3.

Guffey, R. 'William Burroughs: 20th Century Gnostic Visionary'. *New Dawn*. Nov–Dec 2006 99.

Harris, O. *William Burroughs and the Secret of Fascination*. Carbondale and Edwardsville: Southern Illinois University. 2003.

Miles, B. *William Burroughs: El Hombre Invisible*. London: Virgin. 1992.

Murphy, T.S. *Wising Up the Marks: The Amodern William Burroughs*. Berkeley and Los Angeles: University of California. 1997.

Rae, G. 'General Semantics Meets Experimental Literature: The Lifelong Effect of Alfred Korzybski on William S. Burroughs' (given at the Institute of General Semantics's 2009 conference). 2009. Accessed from: http://realitystudio.net/viewtopic.php?t=1097#p9907

Riley, J. 'Playback Hex: William Burroughs and the Magical Objectivity of the Tape Recorder'. *Paranthropology*. 2014 Vol. 5, no.2.

Turnbull, C. *The Forest People*. New York: Simon & Schuster. 1961.

A PSYCHEDELIC TECHNOLOGY:

HOW SET AND SETTING SHAPED THE AMERICAN PSYCHEDELIC EXPERIENCE 1950–1970

IDO HARTOGSOHN

When one looks at the results of 1950s and 1960s LSD research, one finds a peculiar incongruity. Different research groups were giving entirely different and often contradictory accounts of the effects of LSD. One group said LSD was a consciousness expanding agent, leading to enhanced creativity and thought.[1] Yet another group presented results which claimed that LSD caused retardation and poverty of thought.[2] One group claimed LSD enhanced perception, another that it impaired and distorted it.[3, 4] Some researchers were saying that nobody that takes LSD ever wants to repeat the experience again, but others were insisting that every person that had the LSD experience wanted to repeat it again and again.[5] Some regarded LSD as an agent for inducing of psychosis,[6] while others were claiming it would bestow humanity with a new type of sanity.[7]

It was as if researchers were talking about two or more completely different drugs, which produced completely different effects. This situation caused a considerable amount of debate and disagreement as researchers were baffled by the surprising variety of results.

The question this raises is, 'why did the effects of LSD vary so wildly?'. The answer might be obvious to anyone familiar with the dynamics of the psychedelic experience. The reason experimental results with psychedelics varied so markedly was rooted in the set and the setting—the different psychological, social and cultural conditions into which they were inserted.

The set and setting principle, which was proposed by Timothy Leary in the early 1960s,[8] but which actually had roots in some of the 1950s research on the extra-psychopharmacological determinants of drug action.[3, 9, 10] basically claimed that psychedelic drug action, unlike the actions of other types of drugs, was non-specific by nature, and that it was dependent first and foremost on the set of the person having the experience—his personality, preparation, intention and expectation; and on the setting in which the experience was taking place—the physical setting: where did the experience take place; the social setting, with whom; and the cultural setting, in which type of society and culture did this experience take place.

For example, a person who takes a psychedelic in a Buddhist temple, surrounded by monks, with the intention of connecting to some divine reality, is much more likely to have a spiritual experience than a person who undergoes the experience in a hospital room, under the supervision of medical doctors who consider LSD a psychosis mimicking agent.

This explanation, which submits that differences of set and setting were responsible for the divergent results of mid-20th century LSD research, was proposed by a number of prominent LSD investigators of the 1960s, such as Timothy Leary, Willis Harman and Sidney Cohen.[11, 12, 13, 14] It has since gained popularity in the literature, with some authors comparing the story of psychedelic research in the 1960s to the story of the blind men and the elephant, where a group of blind men were asked to touch an elephant and describe its shape. Each of the blind men touched a different part of the elephant's body, therefore giving a completely different description of the animal.[14, 15]

Indeed, when one examines the many forms which LSD research took in the mid-20th century, one finds no fewer than nine different views of LSD related to nine different research agendas. Those include psychotomimetic (psychosis-mimicking) LSD research, psychotherapeutic LSD research, spiritual LSD research, LSD for creativity enhancement, military LSD, special operations LSD research by the CIA, research on LSD and technical innovation, activist LSD, and brain research LSD. The effects of LSD were constructed and shaped differently in each of these contexts. When one analyses the set and setting which was used by different research groups one finds a direct correlation between the type of set and setting used, and the type of results obtained.

This situation, in which the effects of a drug are determined by the environment and conditions in which it is taken, runs completely contrary to basic principles of psychopharmacology. It would seem nonsensical to claim that the effects of a drug change in accordance to the place one takes it, or the group of people one is with. Yet, this is exactly what happens with LSD.

This state of things also raises an intriguing question. One of the most popular and fundamental theories in Science, Technology and Society studies is the theory of the Social Construction of Technology (SCOT). This theory basically claims that the ways in which users perceive a technology cause them to expect different things from it, thus causing the pros and the cons of the technology to be described and worked out differently. The question 'what constitutes a working bike?'—to give the most well-known example in the field—depends on whether you are an elderly person searching for a simple, safe way to move around, or an athletic young man looking to show off his skills while riding a high-wheeler. Socially grounded considerations such as those shaped the ways in which bicycles were understood, designed and built in 19th century England, causing a fundamental shift in the bicycle as a technological artefact.

When we try to apply the SCOT model to the story of LSD in the 1950s and 1960s we find that things go surprisingly beyond the common SCOT model. The structure of a bike might change within a long and complex process in which designers and companies try to answer what they perceive as the expectations of their customers. Nevertheless, however differently one might perceive a bike, its basic attributes—its weight, shape and size

—do not magically change just because one has changed their perception. This, however, was exactly what happened with LSD—the different ways in which people perceived LSD gave rise to fundamental modifications of its effects. LSD is thus a psychedelic technology in the literal sense of the word 'psychedelic' (psyche-mind; delos-manifest). It is a mind-manifesting technology which changes its form in relation to how it is perceived by the mind. LSD recreates itself as a drug and technology in the image of the set and setting into which it is presented, any time it is used.

THE COLLECTIVE SET AND SETTING

What does it mean to have a mind-manifesting technology on your hands? This means that we as a culture bear a responsibility in regards to how we shape that technology. In 1979 Richard Bunce wrote an interesting paper in which he claimed that the rise and fall of the bad trip in the late 1960s and early 1970s was caused by the social and political atmosphere of the time. In a time when government was warning that LSD will fry your brain, give you flashbacks and create genetic damage, and in which people were getting 30 years in prison for smoking a joint, it is no wonder that bad trips became increasingly prevalent, a trend which grew in proportion to the intensity of the drug war and the controversy around LSD. As the 1970s ended and LSD stopped being a political hot potato, so the frequency of bad trips plummeted significantly.[16]

This, in turn, brings us to a crucial and often overlooked aspect of set and setting: the cultural or collective aspect. The discussion on set and setting usually focuses on immediate concerns such as the persons present during the experience, the arrangement of the space, and the user's state of mind before entering the experience. However, there is a crucial element which has been largely absent from the discussion about set and setting over the years. This is the issue of the collective set and setting. In other words, the ways in which cultural conditions predetermine the possible set and setting of an experience.

We can, in fact, speak of two types of set and setting. *An individual set and setting*—the specific and immediate set and setting of an individual psychedelic experience, and then, a second type of set and setting, a collective, cultural set and setting, within which the territory of the individual set and setting is positioned. When we think about it, all the different parameters of set and setting are actually determined to a great extent by society: the personality of a person, his preparation for a psychedelic experience, as well as his intention and expectation upon entering it, are all highly dependent on the society in which he developed and in which he lives. Physical and social setting are also equally dependent on the society and culture.

That such greater cultural structures frame the set and the setting of individual psychedelic experience was already impressively demonstrated by Canadian anthropologist Anthony Wallace in the 1950s.[17] According to Wallace, there were different aspects of cultural attitudes regarding hallucinations which determined their effects. In Western society, for example, the very existence of hallucination was habitually viewed as indicative of mental disease. In many indigenous societies on the other hand, the fact of hallucinating was not considered as reprehensible in itself. Rather, hallucinations were viewed as bearing a meaningful message for the individual and even the society. A person's reaction to his hallucination would thus depend on the way in which the society around them perceives hallucinations, and whether their experience will be accepted and appreciated by the society, or ridiculed, and perhaps even punished.

Wallace noted striking differences in the effects of mescaline on individuals from different cultural groups, comparing its effects on white subjects vs. participators in ceremonies by the Native American Church.

While white users of mescaline exhibited extreme mood swings, alternating between depression, anxiety and euphoria, their Native American counterparts manifested a relative stability of mood, personal satisfaction as well as religious awe. White mescaline users often forsook their social inhibitions, exhibiting sexual and/or aggressive behaviour. They also developed a marked degree of suspiciousness towards others and some other unwelcome mental phenomena such as depersonalisation, split-personality and feeling of meaninglessness.

Native American peyotists, by contrast, remained in good shape and kept up their proper behaviour. Finally, while white subjects showed no therapeutic benefits, their Native American counterparts reported feelings of deep connection with a more meaningful, higher order of existence, and better integration in the community.

This principle, in turn, can teach us a great deal about the story of LSD in mid-20th century research and culture. American society of the 1950s and 1960s underwent great social and cultural changes which in turn shaped how LSD was perceived in the culture. Thus, the conceptions of what LSD is evolved from psychotomimetic conceptions of LSD, to psychotherapeutic and spiritual conceptions, to radical political notions. LSD thus reflected the society and culture into which it was injected. Looking back at the sixties and the fifties in retrospect we can see that many of the phenomena that were considered essential to LSD at the time were actually a reflection of the cultural mood. The strong emphasis on LSD as an agent for torture and psychosis reflected the Cold War mentality of the 1950s, while the 1960s association of psychedelics with hedonism and free sexuality can be considered a reflection of the prominent concerns of the 1960s counterculture.

John Perry Barlow once wrote that the 1960s could be regarded as one long collective trip which was experienced by the American nation upon its confrontation with psychedelics.[18] The concept of collective set-and-setting explains why it is indeed so. The LSD of 1960s America was a unique technological artefact shaped collectively by the unique social and cultural conditions of 1960s America. It is different in its action and properties from the same molecule used in different places and times, a singular collective psychedelic experience which represented the encounter between LSD and the collective set-and-setting conditions of America at the time.

CONCLUSIONS

The story of the role of set and setting in shaping the psychedelic experience of the 1950s and 1960s can teach us significant lessons in an era when psychedelic drug research is making a comeback. First, it can teach us that the effects of psychedelic drugs never exist in a vacuum, but rather they are always mediated by society and culture. Secondly, interpretation matters, and society has responsibility. We can increase the positive effects of psychedelics or we can increase their negative effects. This depends arguably on society, as we saw from the story of the bad trips in the 1960s, which is another reason why the drug war should be abandoned. Finally, it can teach us about what is needed for a successful reintroduction of psychedelics into society. In the decades which have passed since the 1960s, the social controversy around psychedelics has decreased and a greater acceptance of the potential benefit of these agents has been achieved in culture. Creating a more favourable collective set and setting for the reintroduction of psychedelics is key to the fate and the outcome of the current psychedelic renaissance.

References:

1. Harman, W.W., Fadiman, J. 'Selective Enhancement of Specific Capacities Through Psychedelic Training'. In *Psychedelics, The Uses and Implications of Hallucinogenic Drugs.* Aaronson, B., Osmond, H. (eds). New York: Doubleday & Company. 1970. 257–78.

2. Rinkel, M., Deshon, J.H., Hyde, R.W., Solomon, H.C. 'Experimental Schizophrenia-Like Symptoms'. *Am J Psychiatry.* February 1 1952 108(8):572–8.

3. Hyde, R.W. 'Psychological and Social Determinants of Drug Action'. In *Dynamics of Psychiatric Drug Therapy.* 1st ed. Springfield, IL: C.C. Thomas. 1960. 297–315.

4. McGlothlin, W., Cohen, S. 'Long lasting effects of LSD on normals'. *Arch Gen Psychiatry.* November 1 1967 17(5):521–32.

5. Abramson, H.A. *The Use of LSD in Psychotherapy: Transactions of a Conference on D-Lysergic Acid Diethylamide (LSD-25), April 22, 23, and 24,* 1959. Princeton, NJ, New York: Josiah Macy Jr. Foundation. 1960. 316.

6. Hoch, P.H. 'Experimentally Induced Psychoses'. *Am J Psychiatry.* February 1 1951 107(8):607–11.

7. Janiger, O. 'The Use of Hallucinogenic Agents in Psychiatry'. *California Clinician.* 1959 55(7).

8. Leary, T. 'Drugs, Set & Suggestibility'. In *Alteration of Perceptual Consciousness by Drugs.* New York. 1961.

9. Von Felsinger, J.M., Lasagna, L., Beecher, H.K. 'Drug-Induced Mood Changes in Man. II. Personality and Reactions to Drugs'. *JAMA: The Journal of the American Medical Association.* March 26 1955 157(13):1113–9.

10. Slater, P., Morimoto, K., Hyde, R.W. 'The Effect of Group Administration Upon Symptom Formation Under LSD'. *J Nerv Ment Dis.* June 1957 125(2):312–5.

11. Leary, T., Litwin, G., Metzner, R. 'Reactions to Psilocybin Administered in a Supportive Environment'. *J Nerv Ment Dis.* 1963 137:561–73.

12. Metzner, R., Litwin, G., Weil, G.M. 'The Relation of Expectation and Mood to Psilocybin Reactions: A Questionnaire Study'. *Psychedelic Review.* 1966 5.

13. Harman, W.W. 'Some Aspects of the Psychedelic-Drug Controversy'. *Journal of Humanistic Psychology.* April 1 1963 3(2):93–107.

14. Cohen, S.M.D. *The Beyond Within: The LSD Story.* New York: Atheneum. 1970.

15. Fadiman, J. *The Psychedelic Explorer's Guide: Safe, Therapeutic, and Sacred Journeys.* Rochester, Vermont: Park Street Press. 2011. 352.

16. Bunce R. 'Social and Political Sources of Drug Effects: The Case of Bad Trips on Psychedelics'. *Journal of Drug Issues* [Internet]. 1979 (Spring Issue). Available from: http://www.drugtext.org/Control-Over-Intoxicant-Use/social-and-political-sources-of-drugeffects-the-case-of-bad-trips-on-psychedelics.html

17. Wallace, A.F.C. 'Cultural Determinants of Response to Hallucinatory Experience'. *AMA Arch Gen Psychiatry.* July 1 1959 1(1):58–69.

18. Barlow, J.P. 'Foreword'. In *Birth of a Psychedelic Culture: Conversations about Leary, the Harvard Experiments, Millbrook and the Sixties.* Santa Fe, NM: Synergetic Press. 2010.

Funding/Conflicting Interests

I have received no financial support for the research, authorship, and/or publication of this article, and declare that I have no conflicting interests.

ARCHETYPES AND THE COLLECTIVE UNCONSCIOUS: JUNGIAN INSIGHTS INTO PSYCHEDELIC EXPERIENCE

SCOTT J. HILL

When talking about the relevance of Carl Jung's psychology to psychedelic experience, we have a paradox. Considering how little Jung talked explicitly about psychedelic experience, and considering how critical he was of using psychedelic substances, it is paradoxical that so many in the psychedelic community consider Jung an ally. Ann Shulgin, widely regarded as the matriarch of the psychedelic community, is one example. Her work with psychedelic psychotherapy and the shadow is grounded in Jung's psychology.[1] Stanislav Grof, historically the foremost researcher in psychedelic psychotherapy, and arguably the most influential theorist in the field, finds in Jung's psychology a far-reaching correspondence to the domains of psychological experience he has observed during more than five decades of investigation.[2 p187–92]

This appreciation for Jung's psychology is based largely on the relevance of his unique approach to the psyche, his extraordinary personal explorations into the depths of the unconscious, and his mystical sensibility. I'll illustrate these here by showing how Jung's descriptions of archetypes and the collective unconscious provide penetrating insights into psychedelic experience.

JUNG'S CONFRONTATION WITH THE UNCONSCIOUS AND ITS RELATION TO PSYCHEDELIC EXPERIENCE

In the early days of psychedelic research, Carl Jung was invited by Alfred Hubbard to participate in clinical research with mescaline. Jung responded by saying he had never taken mescaline nor given it to another person.[3 p222] Jung eschewed all psychedelic substances because he thought they too quickly and easily open one to the depths of the unconscious, making it impossible to integrate the experience and, worse, possibly pushing a latent psychotic into an acute psychosis. Jung had similar concerns about the analytic form of psychotherapy that he practiced, which had the potential to take a person deep into the unconscious, where things get especially challenging.

So Jung declined the invitation to contribute to mescaline research. But, he said, 'I have at least devoted 40 years of my life to the study of that psychic sphere which is disclosed by said drug; that is the sphere of numinous experiences.'[3 p222] This statement provides the key to understanding the relevance of Jung's psychology to psychedelic experience despite his not having used psychedelics. Jung's study of that numinous sphere of experience was rooted in his personal exploration of the psyche through his dreams, fantasies, and visions—in an arduous process he called his 'confrontation with the unconscious.'[4 ch6] Referring to this process, Jung said:

> The years when I was pursuing my inner images were the most importantinmylife—inthemeverythingessentialwasdecided. [...] The later details are only supplements and clarifications of the material that burst forth from the unconscious, and at first swamped me. It was the prima materia for a lifetime's work.[4 p199]

That is, Jung's whole approach to understanding and explaining the psyche is based on experiences that took him into the same realms that psychedelics can open us to. This similarity is vividly reflected in Jung's *Red Book* paintings, which he created as an aid to and record of his process.

ARCHETYPES AND THE COLLECTIVE UNCONSCIOUS

During his many encounters with the unconscious, Jung became convinced that he was 'obeying a higher will'[4 p177] and that he had encountered an independent psychological force that represented superior insight.[4 p183] And he appreciated that his visions arose from a universal source, what he described as 'the matrix of a mythopoetic imagination which has vanished from our rational age.'[4 p188] For Jung, the universal source of this mythopoetic world was the deepest layers of the unconscious, the collective unconscious. Commenting on prejudices against this mythical world, Jung unintentionally also characterises conventional views against psychedelic experiences:

> It is both tabooed and dreaded, so that it even appears to be a risky experiment or a questionable adventure to entrust oneself to the uncertain path that leads into the depths of the unconscious. It is considered the path of error, of equivocation and misunderstanding. [...] Unpopular, ambiguous, and dangerous, it is a voyage of discovery to the other pole of the world.[4 p188–89]

When Jung speaks of 'the other pole of the world' and 'the depths of the unconscious' and 'the sphere of numinous experiences,' he is alluding to the collective unconscious and the archetypes that dwell there. When seeking to understand psychedelic experiences through a Jungian lens—particularly psychedelic experiences that go beyond sensory and biographical levels to mythical, visionary, and spiritual realms—we can learn a great deal from the way Jung conceives powerful forces that erupt from the depths of the unconscious, forces Jung typically describes as archetypes of the collective unconscious.

Although we shouldn't reify these theoretical concepts, the collective unconscious can be described as that part of the psyche that transmits humanity's shared psychological inheritance. Jung conceives this deepest level of the unconscious as 'combining the characteristics of both sexes, transcending youth and age, birth and death, and [...] having at its command a human experience of one or two million years, practically immortal.'[5 p349 par673] He characterised the collective unconscious as an 'ocean of images and figures which drift into consciousness in our dreams or in abnormal states of mind.'[5 p350 par673]

The concept of an archetype is Jung's theoretical explanation for especially potent unconscious material that can manifest with numinous, or strange and fascinating, effects as dream images and associated emotions or as psychedelic-induced images and associated emotions. Jung cautions that archetypes are quite difficult to understand because the intellect tends to oversimplify their paradoxical nature. Their numinosity and intense emotional charge also make them difficult to comprehend intellectually. Jung concludes, nevertheless, that 'insofar as the archetypes act upon me, they are real and actual to me, even though I do not know what their real nature is.'[4 p352]

Jung described archetypes in different ways as he developed the concept. He first used the term *primordial images* to designate inherited images and themes arising from universal human experiences and expressed through the ages in the world's myths and religions. Consider, for instance, images reflecting the mother, death and rebirth, God, and evil. Later he adopted the term *archetype* to distinguish more explicitly unconscious phenomena and processes, which cannot be observed, from their observable manifestations as, for instance, dream images. Jung emphasised this important distinction when he described the archetype as an inherited *tendency*:

> The term 'archetype' is often misunderstood as meaning a certain definite mythological image or motif. But this would

be no more than a conscious representation. [...] The archetype is, on the contrary, an inherited *tendency* of the human mind to form representations of mythological motifs—representations that vary a great deal without losing their basic pattern. (Jung's emphasis) [6 p228 par523]

The ego, Jung explains, experiences archetypes as completely unexpected and strange; they saturate the conscious mind with 'uncanny forebodings or even with the fear of madness.'[7 p286 par517] Archetypes, Jung said, surface in dreams, hallucinations, and visions with a numinous effect. 'They exert a fascinating and possessive influence upon the conscious mind and can thus produce extensive alterations in the subject.'[8 p70 par110] Archetypes are by no means intrinsically pathological. Indeed, as we shall see, archetypal experiences are potentially healing and transformative. Archetypes become problematic only when we resist their manifestations, or when the ego is overwhelmed by their sudden and unexpected emergence. Nevertheless, Jung had great respect for archetypal experience because the archetypes, he said,

> live in a world quite different from the world outside—in a world where the pulse of time beats infinitely slowly, where the birth and death of individuals count for little. No wonder their nature is strange, so strange that their irruption into consciousness often amounts to a psychosis.[7 p287 par519]

But Jung appreciated the transformative potential of encounters with this strange world—even when those encounters terrify us. As he put it in *Archetypes and the Collective Unconscious* 'It is just the most unexpected, the most terrifyingly chaotic things which reveal a deeper meaning.'[9 p31 par64] It follows that the relationship between the ego and the archetypal unconscious is often initially challenging. Jung poses the problem this way: 'Say you have been very one-sided and lived in a two dimensional world only, behind walls, thinking that you are perfectly safe; then suddenly the sea breaks in: you are inundated by an archetypal world and you are in complete confusion.'[10 p975]

Jung maintains that facing the confusion and fear that can be triggered by this archetypal world can advance psychological transformation. Indeed, Jung believed that 'the most healing, and psychologically the most necessary, experiences are a 'treasure hard to attain,' and its acquisition demands something out of the common.'[11 p82 parl87] In therapeutic practice, Jung observed, this treasure is 'an invasion by archetypal contents'.[11 p82 parl88] There is clinical evidence in the psychedelic therapy literature indicating that experiencing the archetypal unconscious can be healing and transformative.[12, 13, 14, 15, 16]

Jungian-oriented psychiatrist Ronald Sandison, who pioneered LSD therapy in Britain in the early 1950s, describes archetypal experiences as one of three types of psychedelic-induced experiences in LSD therapy. In addition to dream-like hallucinations and reliving forgotten personal memories, Sandison identifies encounters with unconscious images, 'archaic, impersonal images [...] exactly similar in nature to [...] experiences of the collective unconscious which patients undergoing deep analysis experience in their dreams, visual impressions, and fantasies.'[17 p508] Such LSD experiences are accompanied, he adds, 'by a sense of their agelessness and timeless quality which is the hallmark of the great archetypes of the collective unconscious'.[17 p508]

I think Jung epitomises his grasp of psychedelic-induced states of consciousness when he says archetypal experiences impart 'a supernormal degree of luminosity' with emotionally-loaded numinous effects.[18 p436 par841] In *The Red Book*, Jung describes archetypal experiences this way: 'There in the whirl of chaos dwells eternal wonder. Your world begins to become wonderful. Man belongs not only to an ordered world, he also belongs in the wonder-world of his soul.'[19 p264]

THE RELIGIOUS FUNCTION OF THE PSYCHE

The word *soul* in Jung's psychology can often be replaced with the word *psyche*. But the word *soul* here brings attention to the substantial spiritual element in Jung's psychology. This spiritual element is suggested by the Jungian phrase 'the religious function of the psyche,'[20] a phrase that reflects Jung's interest in religious *experience* as opposed to religion—and certainly as opposed to organised Western religions based on authority and belief. Indeed, Jung refreshingly characterises religion as 'the attitude peculiar to a consciousness which has been altered by the experience of the numinosum.'[21 p6]

Jung adopted the idea of the numinosum from Rudolf Otto's[22] use of the term *the numinous* (from *numen*, Latin for divine power). The word *numinous* refers to phenomena having qualities that are experienced as strange, mysterious, and fascinating, and that elicit responses ranging from wonder and awe to dread and terror. For Jung, these phenomena are the archetypes, and he often describes archetypal experience in religious-cum-psychological terms. He has for example characterised archetypal experience in terms of 'holiness,' which for Jung reflects a psychological insight of the highest value, a revelation from beyond the sphere of ego-consciousness that evokes overwhelming awe. It is an illumination emanating from the collective unconscious.[23 p152 par225]

Commenting on the centrality of numinous archetypal experiences in his life and work, Jung wrote that his main interest was the numinous, which he considered the real therapy. 'Inasmuch as you attain to numinous experiences, you are released from the curse of pathology,' he said.[24 p377] Jungian scholar Murray Stein suggests that for Jung the task of approaching the numinous was 'a religious undertaking, a pilgrimage,' and that the attainment to numinous experiences Jung speaks of here refers to religious experiences of a mystical nature.[25 p35]

Despite Jung's objections to using psychedelic substances, some Jungians acknowledge that psychedelic experiences can induce genuine and transformative mystical states of consciousness. Jung himself almost said so in a letter to American psychedelic therapist Betty Eisner in 1957, where he noted that psychedelic drugs such as mescaline can in fact give you certain perceptions and experiences that appear in mystical states. But in the next breath he dismissed psychedelic-induced mystical experiences as 'so-called religious visions' and dangerous substitutes for genuine mystical experiences.[26 p382-383] But Jungian analyst and scholar Lionel Corbett forthrightly recognises the potential psychedelics have to induce authentic spiritual experiences in the form of 'a healing contact with the numinosum.'[27 p65] Corbett saw evidence of this when a woman in his therapeutic practice reported a psychedelic-induced spiritual vision that was directly relevant to her suffering and that was 'extremely helpful.'[27 p65] Jungian analyst Stephen Martin, who is President Emeritus of the Philemon Foundation that funded the publication of Jung's *Red Book*, also recognises that psychedelically mediated encounters with the unconscious can be authentically transformative. Martin unequivocally acknowledges 'the potential value of the psychedelic experience as a bona fide agent in personal transformation.'[28 p258] The views of Corbett and Martin are no doubt shared by many Jungians, although the extent of this agreement is difficult to judge given the risk that still exists for mental health professionals to publically acknowledge the transformative potential of psychedelics.

THE ISSUE OF PSYCHOLOGISING RELIGIOUS EXPERIENCES

Jung has been criticised for 'psychologising' religious experiences by reducing their objective metaphysical reality to intrapsychic experiences. Although this is a complex issue, I am becoming increasingly convinced that this criticism reflects a limited understanding of Jung's approach to archetypes, the collective unconscious, synchronicity, and the psyche as a whole, in all its mysterious depth.

Jung's approach to religious experience was complex and continued to develop over his lifetime. In *C.G. Jung's Psychology of Religion and Synchronicity*,[29] Robert Aziz classifies the religious or spiritual aspects of Jung's psychology into two models: the intrapsychic model and the synchronistic model. Aziz argues that Jung's intrapsychic approach to religious experience does reduce religious experiences to psychological experiences, as evidenced by statements like this one by Jung:

[Psychology] treats all metaphysical claims and assertions as mental phenomena, and regards them as statements about the mind and its structure that derive ultimately from certain unconscious dispositions. [i.e. archetypes.]. It does not consider [metaphysical claims and assertions] to be absolutely valid or even capable of establishing a metaphysical truth.[30 p476 par760]

Such statements clearly reduce religious experiences and content to unconscious projections. But such statements also reflect Jung's avowed role as psychologist and scientist. That is, they reflect Jung's principled refusal to take a position—one way or the other—on the metaphysical nature of religious experiences and content. In the same paragraph just quoted, Jung acknowledges that it is possible that our psyches are manifesting extrapsychic realities.[30 p476 par760] So even though Jung is adamant that the psyche *mediates* religious experiences, as a scientist of his time he simply refused to affirm metaphysical realities beyond what he could empirically observe. This is an understandable and justifiable agnostic stance, which by definition neither confirms nor denies extrapsychic realities.

But clearly Jung was more than a scientist of his time; and despite his probable fear of the charge of mysticism, he occasionally revealed his openness to there being more—much more—to religious experience than he could confirm scientifically. In his conclusion to 'A Psychological Approach to the Dogma of the Trinity,' Jung states:

These considerations have made me extremely cautious in my approach to the further metaphysical significance that may possibly underlie archetypal statements. There is nothing to stop their ultimate ramifications from penetrating to the very ground of the universe. We alone are the dumb ones if we fail to notice it. Such being the case, I cannot pretend to myself that the object of archetypal statements has been explained and disposed of merely by our investigation of its psychological aspects.[23 p200 par295]

But most significantly, as Aziz shows, Jung's synchronicity theory throws an entirely new light on his psychology of religious experience and his concept of the archetype. Jung conceived of synchronicity as a meaningful parallel between inward, psychological, events and outward, environmental, events that are not causally related. Such events are understood as manifestations of an acausal order that transcends time and space.[29] [p2] Indeed, Jung's observations of synchronistic occurrences led him to a new view of reality. His observations led him in particular to an expanded model of the archetypes, a radical re-visioning of archetypes as psycho-physical ('psychoid') phenomena with numinous or mystical qualities that transcend time, space, and causality, manifesting in both the individual psyche and in nature.

Since psyche and matter are contained in one and the same world, and moreover are in continuous contact with one another and ultimately rest on irrepresentable, *transcendental factors* [i.e. archetypes], it is not only possible but fairly probable, even, that psyche and matter are two different aspects of one and the same thing. (emphasis added)[31] [p215 par418]

With these theoretical developments, Jung had clearly gone beyond a strictly intrapsychic view of the archetypes to a holistic view of the world and our psychological existence within it, a view reflected in his use of the Latin term, the *unus mundus*, the unitary world. The idea of the *unus mundus*, Jung explains,

is founded on the assumption that the multiplicity of the empirical world rests on an underlying unity, and that not two or more fundamentally different worlds exist side by side. [...] Rather, everything divided and different belongs to one and the same world.[32] [p537–538 par767]

As Aziz suggests, Jung's theoretical progression from seeing archetypes as strictly intrapsychic phenomena to seeing them as transcendental factors in a unitary world has clear metaphysical implications.[29 p174] Jung himself seems to tacitly concede this in his principal essay on synchronicity. Referring to the psychoid nature of the archetypes, Jung writes:

> We are so accustomed to regard meaning as a psychic process or content that it never enters our heads to suppose that it could exist outside the psyche. [...] If, therefore, we entertain the hypothesis that one and the same (transcendental) meaning might manifest itself simultaneously in the human psyche and in the arrangement of an external and independent event, we at once come into conflict with the conventional scientific and epistemological views.[18 p482 par915]

It is fair to say that the entire movement of Jung's personal exploration of the unconscious and the overall development of his thought and his approach to the psyche came into conflict with conventional scientific and epistemological views. One can find evidence of this throughout his vast body of work, but I'll close here, where Jung writes:

> In our ordinary mind we are in the worlds of time and space and within the separate individual psyche. In the state of the archetype we are in the collective psyche, in a world-system whose space-time categories are relatively or absolutely abolished. [...] We are not capable of functioning in a four dimensional system at will; it only can happen to us. Our intellectual means reach only as far as archetypal experiences, but within that sphere, we are not the motors, we are the moved objects.[33 p399]

For those of us looking for a deeper understanding of psychedelic experience, an understanding that goes beyond the conventional, we are surely fortunate that Carl Jung had the intelligence and the courage to descend into that other pole of the world and discover the realms of archetypal experience.

Sources:

1. Shulgin, A. 'The new psychotherapy: MDMA and the shadow'. In *Psychoactive Sacramentals: Essays on entheogens and religion*. Roberts, T. (ed). San Francisco: Council on Spiritual Practices. 2001. 197–204.

2. Grof, S. *Beyond the Brain: Birth, Death and Transcendence in Psychotherapy*. Albany, NY: SUNY Press. 1985.

3. Jung, C.G. Letter to A. M. Hubbard. *C.G. Jung Letters*, Vol. 2. Princeton University Press. 1975.

4. Jung, C.G. Memories, Dreams, Reflections. New York: Vintage Books. 1963.

5. Jung, C.G. 'Basic postulates of analytical psychology'. *The Collected Works of C.G. Jung*, Vol. 8. Princeton University Press. 1969.

6. Jung, C.G. 'Symbols and the interpretation of dreams'. *The Collected Works of C.G. Jung*, Vol.18. London: Routledge. 1977.

7. Jung, C.G. 'Conscious, unconscious, and individuation'. *The Collected Works of C.G. Jung*, Vol. 9, Part I. Princeton University Press. 1969.

8. Jung, C.G. 'The personal and collective (or transpersonal) unconscious'. *The Collected Works of C.G. Jung*, Vol. 7. Princeton University Press. 1966.

9. Jung, C.G. 'Archetypes and the collective unconscious'. *The Collected Works of C.G. Jung*, Vol. 9, Part I. Princeton University Press. 1969.

10. Jung, C.G. 'Nietzsche's Zarathustra: Notes of the seminar given in 1934-1939', Vol. 2. Princeton University Press. 1988.

11. Jung, C.G. 'Psychotherapy and a philosophy of life'. *The Collected Works of C.G. Jung*, Vol. 16. Princeton University Press. 1966.

12. Cutner, M. 'Analytic work with LSD-25'. *Psychiatric Quarterly*. 1959 33(4):715–757.

13. Sandison, R. *A Century of Psychiatry, Psychotherapy and Group Analysis: A search for integration*. London: Jessica Kingsley. 2001.

14. Grof, S. *LSD Psychotherapy*. Sarasota, FL: Multidisciplinary Association for Psychedelic Studies. 2001.

15. Papaspyrou, M. 'In search of the philosopher's stone'. In *Neurotransmissions: Essays on psychedelics from Breaking Convention*. King, D., Luke, D., Sessa, B., Adams, C., Tollan, A. (eds). London: Strange Attractor Press. 2015.

16. Hill, S. *Confrontation with the Unconscious: Jungian depth psychology and psychedelic experience*. London: Muswell Hill Press. 2013.

17. Sandison, R. 'Psychological aspects of the LSD treatment of the neuroses'. *Journal of Mental Science*. 1954 100:508–515.

18. Jung, C.G. 'Synchronicity: An acausal connecting principle'. *The Collected Works of C.G. Jung*, Vol. 8. Princeton University Press. 1969.

19. Jung, C.G. *The Red Book: Liber Novus*. London & New York: Norton. 2009.

20. Corbett, L. *The Religious Function of the Psyche*. New York: Brunner-Routledge. 1996.

21. Jung, C.G. *Psychology and Religion*. New Haven, CT: Yale University Press. 1966.

22. Otto, R. *The Idea of the Holy*. New York: Oxford University Press. 1958.

23. Jung, C.G. 'A psychological approach to the dogma of the trinity'. *The Collected Works of C.G. Jung*, Vol. 11. Princeton University Press. 1969.

24. Jung, C.G. Letter to P.W. Martin, *C.G. Jung Letters*, Vol. 1. Princeton: Princeton University Press. 1975.

25. Stein, M. 'On the importance of numinous experience in the alchemy of individuation'. In *The Idea of the Numinous*. Casement, A., Tacey, D., (eds). London. Routledge. 2006.

26. Jung, C.G. Letter to B. G. Eisner. *C.G. Jung Letters*, Vol. 2. Princeton University Press. 1975.

27. Corbett, L. 'Varieties of numinous experience: the experience of the sacred in therapeutic process'. In *The Idea of the Numinous*. Casement, A., Tacey, D., (eds). London. Routledge. 2006.

28. Martin, S.A. *'Review of Confrontation with the unconscious: Jungian depth psychology and psychedelic experience*, Scott J. Hill'. *Journal of Transpersonal Psychology*. 2014 46(2):257–259.

29. Aziz, R. *C.G. Jung's Psychology of Religion and Synchronicity*. Albany, NY: SUNY Press. 1990.

30. Jung, C.G. 'Psychological commentary on the Tibetan book of the great liberation'. *The Collected Works of C.G. Jung*, Vol. 11. Princeton University Press. 1969.

31. Jung, C.G. 'On the nature of the psyche'. *The Collected Works of C.G. Jung*, Vol. 8. Princeton University Press. 1969.

32. Jung, C.G. 'The conjunction'. *The Collected Works of C.G. Jung*, Vol. 14. Princeton University Press. 1970.

33. Jung, C.G. Letter to Stephen Adams. *C.G. Jung Letters*, Vol. 2. Princeton University Press. 1975.

ALTERED STATES OF UNCONSCIOUS: A QUESTION OF ELF AND SAFETY

WILL ROWLANDSON

Entities exist in many realms. There are the realms of the dead, the realms of dreams, and the realms of the imagination. There are also the spirits of animals, the spirits of the Earth and solar system and stars, and the angelic stellar intelligences. There are spirits of each species of plant or mushroom, each with its own way of being, its own way of seeing and experiencing the world, of participating in the whole.—Rupert Sheldrake[1]

An abstract, cognizant entity may be impossible to know directly because of the complexity of the multidimensional spheres of the world soul. But when the entity structure descends, diffusing down through spirit, it becomes increasingly simple and develops more and more into cognitive forms that belong to the human mind in its evolutionary resonance with morphogenetic fields. At these lower levels, the entity is forced into representations that are culturally dependent such as faeries, dakinis, elementals, and so on.—Ralph Abraham[1]

In all times and all places, with the possible exception of Western Europe for the past two hundred years, a social commerce between human beings and various types of discarnate entities, or non-human intelligences, was taken for granted.—Terence McKenna[1]

As the Trialogians indicate above, the pesky pixies and naughty numens just won't go away. They have been with us for millennia and they will remain with us, one assumes, for millennia. Ghostly stick beings and therianthropes adorn our ancestors' cave walls. St Paul admonished the Corinthians to reject demons and pagan idolatry, and Christianity has ever since had troubled relationships with sprites and spirits, fairies, elves and goblins. Ghouls, grotesques and gargoyles leer from mediaeval church towers and portals as both threat and appeal. Chaucer's Wife of Bath sings of the lost time of Arthur, when: 'All was this land fulfild of fayerye. / The elf-queene, with hir joly compaignye.' Shakespeare's Puck, the fairy king Oberon's jester, is called by a fairy 'that shrewd and knavish sprite / Call'd Robin Goodfellow', or, as Puck calls himself, 'that merry wanderer of the night'. Elizabeth I [who incidentally was born and lived on the grounds where the University of Greenwich, home of BC, now stands. Ed.] was likened to the Fairy Queen, whilst her magus-spy John Dee rapped with angels. Girls in pinafores frolic with garden fairies in tricksy Victorian photographs. Robert Louis Stevenson thanked the Brownies for providing him with his stories, such as *Jekyll and Hyde*. Alien greys gaze passively from 20th century ufology; and so it goes on in an endless list across cultures and ages.

Jung's 1958 essay *Flying Saucers: A Modern Myth of Things Seen in the Skies*[2] is a penetrating study of the phenomenon of UFOs, concentrating not on questions of the material status of the flying saucers—where do they come from, what are they, how do they fly, etc. —but on why are they appearing in our skies? What does their appearance suggest about those who witness them or pay an interest in them? He appraised their circular form as mandalas, as symbols of mankind's yearning for the sacred; as psychic effect, arising out of the de-sacralised barren landscape of the modern, technological, atomic, Cold War era. His question in essence was: Why flying saucers—why now?

I borrowed Jung's model[3] to consider the phenomenon of crop formations, transcending the perplexing debate about who made them (are they made by humans and therefore 'fake', or by some other agency and therefore 'real'?) to consider what they mean, how they are approached, how they appear to trigger anomalous experiences in both those who make them and those who chart them. I also considered their mandala nature and their evocation of collective yearning for the sacred. Why crop circles—why now?

I followed a similar method[4] to consider the meaningful appearance of ayahuasca beyond its traditional cultural environment, considering the reintegration of the daimonic and the indigenous, and the implications of plant consciousness in our rigid technological age. Why ayahuasca—why now?

The story now leads me to consider the reappearance of elfin entities in the collective imagination, in particular those elves encountered through psilocybin and DMT. Why elves—why now?

Such a myth-oriented approach is not to belittle the heuristic steps taken by many scholars to consider, precisely, the ontological status of psychedelic elves. It is important to base investigation on where these entities dwell—what realities, what dimensions, inner or outer, material or imaginary—and to consider the nature of their autonomy and their relationship with the psyche of the voyager.

Terence McKenna[1] posits three distinct bases from which to evaluate the ontological status of the elves: 'The first option is that these entities are rare, but physical, and that they have identities somewhere between the coelacanths and Bigfoot'. The second option he calls 'the Jungian position' citing Jung's 'autonomous fragments of psychic energy that have temporarily escaped from the controlling power of the ego'. His third possibility, 'the most interesting, but the one fraught with argumentative pitfalls, is that these entities are (1) nonphysical and (2) autonomous in their existence in some sense' (93–4).

Peter Meyer, in a pioneering article,[5] isolates three distinct fields from which to address the questions about the DMT elves: the neuropharmacological (what is happening to the brain?), the phenomenological (what are trippers reporting?), and the ontological (what is the nature of being of these entities and their environment?). He articulates eight possible responses to this final question, amongst which that the elves are: (i) simple hallucination, (ii) 'independently-existing intelligent entities' from a 'parallel or higher dimension', (iv) a view of reality from the reptilian mind (DMT as an ancient, pre-mammalian neurotransmitter), (vi) the souls of the dead, and (viii) 'probes from an extraterrestrial or even an extradimensional species, sent out to make contact with organisms such as ourselves.'

Variations and further hypotheses have been offered by countless others, as documented by Graham St John in his recent cultural history of DMT, *Mystery School in Hyperspace*,[6] ranging from mere hallucination occasioned by neurochemical perturbation to encounters with hyperspatial ETs. How are we to navigate such complex and contradictory positions?

My intuition is to consider each possibility equally plausible and equally valid, basing my method upon sympathy for the *imaginal* nature of reality: dreams and visions are no mere hallucination; they are coded narratives connected symbolically to the subject and are therefore, however vague materially, not unreal. Might the elves be one day classified within our taxonomical schema, like the coelacanth? It is unlikely, but giant squids—the mythical kraken—have been hauled up from the depths. The coelacanth itself is a mythic beast—a living fossil forgotten by evolution from the cretaceous. As Borges reminds us, a lion is both animal and symbol. Myth and reality are always intertwined.

McKenna dismisses the Jungian position as 'the mentalist-reductionist approach to discarnate entities,' predicating his judgement, I imagine, on the understanding that Jung considered the psyche essentially interior and non-material (his *adlib* citation of Jung is, I surmise, from Jung's 1921 work *Psychological Types*). As such, he was likely not aware of Jung's vivid accounts of encounters with strikingly autonomous psychic intelligences in *The Red Book*,[7] published a decade after McKenna's death.

In this dazzling illustrated book, Jung dialogues with the prophet Elijah and John the Baptist's nemesis, Salome. Jung is troubled by their radical autonomy and declares: 'I can hardly reckon you as being part of my soul [...] Therefore I must separate you and Salome from my soul and place you among the daimons' (357). Such is the autonomous nature of Salome and Elijah that when Jung confronts them and suggests that 'You are the symbol of the most extreme contradiction', Elijah retorts: 'We are real and not symbols' (246). Later, Elijah returns to this matter and explains: 'You may call us symbols for the same reason that you can also call your fellow men symbols, if you wish to. But we are just as real as your fellow men. You invalidate nothing and solve nothing by calling us symbols' (249).

Elijah's response is tremendous, as he urges Jung to understand that we are all daimonic beings, forever encountered symbolically by others, forever encountering others symbolically.

Not everything in *The Red Book* is as clear as this response, and I feel its impact lies with Jung's bewilderment when confronted with figures of such overwhelming autonomy. Hence his ultimate desire to tell them that they are not real because he is dreaming them. His guru figure, Philemon is, by Jung's own account, far more of an individuated soul than he is. He is, indeed, a wise old man.

Jung clearly understood in his dealings with Philemon, Salome and Elijah that there is something *utterly* beyond our consciousness that is nevertheless part of our consciousness. He learns to feel that they are real because he dreams them. Elijah seems quite peeved, rebuking Jung for doubting his sovereignty.

Such is the sense of the trip reports in Strassman's *DMT: The Spirit Molecule*[8] where subjects describe stumbling into an elfin engagement, rather than in any way 'inventing' or 'imagining' the encounter.

Such is the atmosphere of Swedenborg's spiritual adventures. The angels he dialogues with were busy prior to his arrival and will be busy once he departs. They do not appear to surge into existence through his creative imagination any more than his friends in London, Stockholm or Amsterdam do. Swedenborg would not be so rude as to suggest to them that he was somehow their creator.

I can illustrate this drama: when in Paris you ask a passer-by directions, yet while she points down the street to indicate, you stare at her wide-eyed and you ask her 'are you real? Am I dreaming you? Are you a fiction, a creature of my imagination?' The chances are you will get lost.

You have an appointment with the doctor, to seek healing for your sore knee. Yet while she is diagnosing the ailment and considering a treatment you ask, astonished, *'what is your ontological status?'*. My sense is that your knee would not heal.

So if you seek healing from a saint or from Christ or from the fairies by the well or the pixies at the waterfall, there is no point in asking for healing but apologising for knowing that they're not *really* there, that they can't *really* help. How rude!

Saint Fulano, I seek your help!
(but I secretly know you're just a statue).

What kind of help do you want? You won't get much help from a mere statue. No—you must invest! This shit's real. Stop the chatter. Stop interrupting yourself when asking for guidance or healing by allowing yourself to see it as make-believe. (Although such a strategy may very effectively be employed to shrivel up a monster—tell him he is simply make-believe!)

Jung likewise moved from asking whether he had dreamt of his dead father or whether his father visited him in his dreams, to concerning himself with what his father had to say.

What does a dead relative have to say?
What are the elves saying?
What do we seek with them and they with us?

This is a well-reported feature of ayahuasca encounters: don't be so astonished by us, say the elves, the serpent, the jaguar or the luminous woman, listen to what we have to say...

And so don't quiz the elf about its ontological status, especially knowing its trickster nature. Elf today pixie tomorrow. They're self-transforming. You can't catch an elf in a box.

Listen to the voices, don't pathologise them.
But don't idolise them.

Graham St John suggests:[9] 'perhaps it is not what these entities are or where they come from that ultimately matters, but what these anomalies can do for us. Rather than fixating on where they come from, it appears more fruitful to explore the meaning and implications of their message, whether on a scale of personal growth or consciousness evolution.' Indeed; and following his suggestion we may ask: what do the elves *mean*? Why elves—why now?

Elves are not angels. They are tricksters; mercurial, hermetic, inhabiting crossroads and crooked trees and standing stones on the moonlit moorland.

Certain states of consciousness are required in order to engage with the elves. They appear in reverie and in vision, in the flickers of the fire, in the shadows of the twilit woodland, in the ripples of the stream, in the moment of enchantment reading a child a fairy story. 'And so Snow White ate the poisoned apple and died and the dwarves laid her in a glass casket...'

There will be no encounter through tough-minded rational analysis. Let go—circle awhile in the lazy eddies of space-time. Drift into reverie. Be enchanted.

They can lure us off the path. The lone Irish tippler in so many of the stories collected by William Butler Yeats staggers home along the track and is enticed into the mire to join the fairy dance.

Treat them respectfully and they'll protect you and give you a boon—perhaps the gift of music and dance, perhaps psychic strength to accept change, perhaps simply a good story to tell on long winter nights. Do we not thank Santa and his elves for the presents by leaving a mince pie and a nip of sloe gin? In Asturias, in northern Spain, the domestic *trasgu* (I think a distant cousin of the Leprechaun) will steal things if you do not leave him a bit of cake or a drop of cider from time to time.

Treat the elves disrespectfully and they'll disrespect you, tripping you up, like the A.A. Milne poem of Brave Sir Botany who falls in the village fishpond in his fine armour. Shakespeare's fairy asks Puck: 'are not you he / That frights the maidens of the villagery [...] Mislead night wanderers, laughing at their harm?' The elves in Borges' *Book of Imaginary Beings* steal cattle and, occasionally, steal children.

Neglect poor Santa and he may neglect you. What! No presents?

There are the gremlins in the machine, knocking out parts of the ordered system, rerouting, jarring. We get angry – *fucking computer's frozen again* – but can we see the freeze as an opportunity to question the importance of the job we were doing on the computer? Need we be staring at a screen? Is that touchy unsent email necessary? Is it not the moment to breathe and stretch and walk and make a cup of tea?

Gremlins, like elves, are elements of change. Change can be tough, but change can be enriching. You see to be lured off the path is to be pulled out of a rut... to be enticed into enchantment... to be spun out of the routine.

Elves are routine-busters. They are resistant to rigid structures of control and order. Simply discussing elves is a heterodox act—*elves? What do you mean, elves? You mean the wee beasties in fairy stories? You can't be serious!*

There are McKenna's machine elves, who chant Syd Barrett's 'another way for gnomes to say, hoooooorrrrrraaaaaayyyyyy', and who giggle and fold in and out of space-time, saying 'do what we are doing', which is throwing about wobbly language balls. Play!

There are the silent Hattifattener-like witnesses I have seen whilst lying bemushroomed in a yellow tent in the woods on a crisp autumn afternoon, who simply hang in there, abiding. Old like the hills.

There is the elfin king himself—the Green Man—hiding in plain sight right up against the throne of ecclesiastical authority, reminding us all that the straight lines and ordered symmetry of our temples will one day be ivy-clad, home for birds and beetles. No power of sword and scripture can unsettle the Green Man. He abides.

There are the white elves of *The Lord of the Rings*, sombre and severe, but capable of powerful magic. Well they need to be powerful, faced with the horror of Mordor. I can understand why they're sombre. Sometimes it is necessary to fight steel with steel, ugliness with righteous indignation.

Elves are sneaky and mischievous. Well, is that not cunning and resourceful? If we are keen to resist rigid structures of control and order, we likewise need to be cunning and resourceful. They are allies for those resisting injustice, brutality and aggression, not least because the elves can be unjust, brutal and aggressive.

Keep your wits about you. Don't abandon your power of critical perception. Today, amidst the goblin market of religions, ideologies and slogans, we must keep our wits about us. There are forces keen to ensnare us, trap us and trip us. The elves teach us to keep alert by trapping and tripping us. Don't be coerced. Don't be coerced, especially by elves.

They can help you in a fight. But they might bite you too. The elves, I think, resist playfully yet earnestly the ravages of capital modernity. Elves would not renew Trident. Elves would not frack. It is not in elfin spirit to bulldoze forests, to poison streams, to massacre the buffalo and the whale; not in the elfin spirit to bulldoze cultures, not in the elfin spirit to annihilate.

But it might be in goblin nature. Were your encounters with elves or goblins? How to distinguish? Many goblins have flipped and followed the trickster dynamic to its hurtful rather than healing ends.

They begin innocuously enough, like the eerie Hobgoblin in Tove Jansson's *Finn Family Moomintroll*,[10] who wanders the universe with his flying panther, looking for the King's Ruby, and whose top hat causes chaos in the Moominhouse by transforming anything put in it into weird creatures.

Or the goblins of Brian Froud and Allen Lee's *Faeries*, who are trickster and sprightly yet never malevolent. Or the goblins of Christina

Rossetti's poem 'Goblin Market', who entice with fruity bounty: 'Apples and quinces, Lemons and oranges, Plump unpeck'd cherries, Melons and raspberries, [...] All ripe together, In summer weather,' but who are quick to anger and quick to avenge.

Or the naughty Goblins in the *Noddy* tales, Sly and Gobbo. In one story they steal Noddy's car and crash it—poor Noddy. But they provide the plot to so many of the stories. They're integral to the fragile geometry of Toyland. They create the friction that Noddy's nice friends just somehow fail to create. Big-Ears the brownie and Tessie Bear, are, well, just a little dull. Sly and Gobbo would be fun to get drunk with. They were the childhood friends your parents wanted you to avoid. They're rude and impolite—they'll lead you astray—they're troublemakers. They're unpleasant, but they're not Orks.

Orks are goblins. They're savage. They win battles. They cut down trees. They clear the forests in order to make more Orks. They multiply through destruction. They buy into the ideologies of Sauron —his hideous promises of power and the indulgence of material desire. That's the nature of the Ork, and even the gentle Samwise finds the courage to fight them. Tolkien's Orks and Goblins are brothers in vileness, and he attributes to them man's capacity for vileness: 'It is not unlikely,' Tolkien wrote, 'that they invented some of the machines that have since troubled the world, especially the ingenious devices for killing large numbers of people at once, for wheels and engines and explosives always delighted them.'

Goblins are capable of burning the trees and poisoning the wells. Swedenborg relates that we attract souls as to our own disposition. We must be alert to our congress with goblins. Never trust a goblin. Beware goblin tricks.

Just because you meet an elf it doesn't mean he's not a goblin. Just because you meet a goblin it doesn't mean he's not an Ork. If an Ork, what then? Remember that there is Ork in us all. Are you acting Orkishly? Have you been an Ork lately?

Yet neither is it in the elfin spirit to bring mankind together in one great shining peaceful harmony. No heavenly circles of light and purity and freshly laundered white clothes. No—the elves are more earthy, more mischievous, more tied to the dirty truths of embodied existence.

The elves are the allies for those who grow in the shadows of the moonlight, for those who groove the grooves of an old oak. I see the elves engaged in a discourse of environmental consciousness. This is a voice of enchantment.

'The elves and gnomes,' McKenna tells us, 'are there to remind us that, in the matter of understanding the self, we have yet to leave the playpen in the nursery of ontology.'

Right—we are like children again, asking whether fairies are real, not like fairy-story real but really real... like you and me. We are plunged again into childhood naiveté, questioning openly the ideological underpinnings of consensual reality. Naive perhaps, enchanting, certainly. For our society is set on a pathway of disenchantment. The problems we face are the result of de-sacralisation and disenchantment.

Ugly architecture, polluted rivers, dull tomatoes, boring TV, hurt and pain and suffering, corruption, torture. Torture! There are people who torture, people trained to torture. Which numens are they evoking? Perhaps the goblins.

We know the natural ethic of our heart. We know how to discern the tricks that heal from the tricks that harm—but sometimes we need to re-learn how to discern—how to listen to that natural ethic of our heart.

Ralph Abraham, like many others, suggests that entities garb themselves in the trappings of the age. These multidimensional grinning fractal machine elves may have lost their leather jerkins and acorn hats, but they retain their elfin nature.

Elves appear today amidst the mycelial internetworks of communication connecting folk across the globe. Such is the presence of Terence McKenna in this hyper-cyber-space that the elves are likely to dress as he depicted and favour singing Syd Barrett over fiddling a jig.

As with every previous cultural dynamic, elves and similar entities are upsetting the established patterns of reality. They will not be pinned down, however consensually they manifest, and however meticulously we search in the micro-circuitry of the mind. McKenna claimed that there is something differentiating the machine elves from traditional elves—that they are visible to anyone who trips the tryptamines. But not everyone does. Not everyone hunts the high hills for the Yeti nor plunges the depths of Loch Ness. The reports can still be dismissed as frivolous fancy.

The elves unsettle; they are unsettling. They enchant and yet ensnare. They sparkle in sunlit beauty then leer ravenously in fluorescent goblin wickedness. They teach through tricks, teaching adeptness, alertness, discernment, plant-like adaptability, patience. They play the sweetest music, drawing you through the dancing flames, through the rippling water, through the sun-speckled green branches into the lushest reverie... and then steal your phone.

Next time, don't take your phone.

Sources:

Abraham, R., McKenna, T., Sheldrake, R. *Trialogues at the Edge of the West: Chaos, Creativity, and the Resacralization of the World*. Bear & Company. 1992.

Jung, C.G. 'Flying Saucers: A Modern Myth of Things Seen in the Sky' CW 10: *Civilization in Transition*. 1958 307–437.

Rowlandson, W. 'Crop formations as psychoid manifestation. Borrowing Jung's Analysis of UFOs to Approach the Phenomenon of the Crop Circle'. *Paranthropology: Journal of Anthropological Approaches to the Paranormal*. 2011 Vol. 2 no. 4: 42–59.

Rowlandson, W. 'Ayahuasca, ecology and indigeneity'. In *Neurotransmissions: Essays on Psychedelics from Breaking Convention*. Adams, C., et al. (eds). Strange Attractor Press. 2015. 161–173.

Meyer, P. 'Apparent communication with discarnate entities induced by dimethyltryptamine (DMT)'. In Lyttle, T. (ed). *Psychedelics*. New York: Barricade Books. 1994. 161–203.

St John, G. *Mystery School in Hyperspace: A Cultural History of DMT*. Evolver Editions. 2015.

Jung, C.G. *The Red Book: Liber Novus*. Shamdasani, S. (ed). London: Norton. 2009.

Strassman, R. *DMT: The Spirit Molecule: A Doctor's Revolutionary Research into the Biology of Near-Death and Mystical Experiences*. Park Street Press. 2001.

St John, G., Davis, E. 'The Mystery of DMT: A Talk with Graham St John'. 2016. Reality Sandwich. http://realitysandwich.com/319198/mystery-school-in-hyperspace

Jansson, T. *Finn Family Moomintroll*. London: Puffin Books. 1973.

RANDOM SELECTIONS: FROM RESEARCH TOOLS TO RESEARCH CHEMICALS

DAVID E. NICHOLS

The overall structure of this talk will include entactogens, and how we defined them; how we studied new substances in the laboratory without using human testing; and finally some derivatives of LSD that helped us to understand further some of the important structural features of ergoline type psychedelics.

It should first of all be noted that all of the classic serotonergic hallucinogens, entactogens, and most psychostimulants target specific brain receptors or monoamine reuptake carriers. The natural transmitters serotonin, dopamine, and norepinephrine are all essentially 'arylethylamines', meaning that they are an aromatic ring system two carbon atoms removed from a basic amino group. Thus, to a certain extent, what we discovered with certain molecules was relevant to biological target sites for these three neurotransmitters.

For our work, which was all preclinical (meaning not in humans) we studied three principle pharmacological classes of drugs. First, psychostimulants are drugs that increase locomotor activity in rodents, then can be self-administered in rodents, they also are active in a behavioural model called conditioned place preference (CPP), which measures how rewarding (or aversive) a particular drug is, and if one implants a microdialysis probe into specific areas of the brain, psychostimulants generally increase extracellular concentrations of dopamine. These drugs can lead to dependence and addiction.

The second class we studied were the entactogens. These drugs have a pharmacology that is very similar to the psychostimulants, except that a major component of their action is the release of neuronal serotonin from axon terminals, which can also be measured using in vivo microdialysis in rodents. Entactogens such as MDMA have low dependence liability, but can have serious cardiovascular side effects. Although many people believe that MDMA and other entactogens only release neuronal serotonin, in fact they also release both dopamine and norepinephrine, which likely are major players in the stimulant properties of entactogens.

Finally, we studied hallucinogens (psychedelics). These drugs have high affinity and are agonists at a type of brain serotonin receptor called the 5-HT2A receptor. Besides measuring their in vitro receptor effects, we trained rats to discriminate injections of LSD from saline in a two-lever drug discrimination task.

When MDMA first became popular, some characterised it as 'just another substituted hallucinogenic amphetamine.' In the presentation I highlighted the fact that MDMA could not have that pharmacology for three important reasons (Nichols 1986, Nichols, Hoffman et al. 1986). First, hallucinogenic amphetamines possess their greatest activity in the R or levo stereochemistry, whereas the more active enantiomer of MDMA has the S or dextro configuration. Second, when a methyl group is added to the basic nitrogen of an hallucinogenic amphetamine, activity is abolished. By contrast, MDMA has an N-methyl group and is active. Finally, if the alpha-methyl of an hallucinogen amphetamine is extended to an alpha-ethyl moiety, activity is also completely lost. Yet, the alpha-ethyl homolog of MDMA (MBDB) retains entactogenic activity. Thus, entactogens can be differentiated from hallucinogen amphetamines by the fact that (1) their (+)-isomers are more active; (2) they have N-methyl (or ethyl) groups; and (3) entactogenic activity is retained in compounds with an alpha-ethyl moiety. These points are illustrated in the first figure opposite.

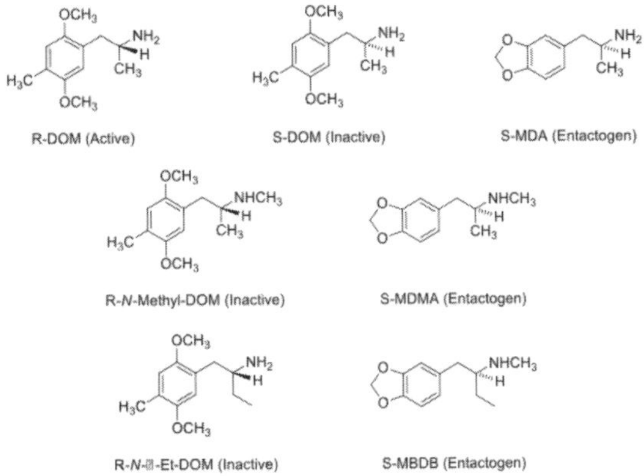

R-DOM (Active)   S-DOM (Inactive)   S-MDA (Entactogen)

R-N-Methyl-DOM (Inactive)   S-MDMA (Entactogen)

R-N-ẞ-Et-DOM (Inactive)   S-MBDB (Entactogen)

In our structure-activity studies, we identified the shape, or 'conformation' that MDMA adopted at its biological target sites, presumably the monoamine uptake carriers. By constraining the side chain of MDMA into either a five or six membered ring, we could demonstrate that only one conformation had MDMA-like activity (Nichols, Brewster et al. 1990). One of those compounds, MDAI, later appeared on the recreational chemical market. In the figure below, the numbers below the structures are the ED50 values for the drugs when tested in rats trained to discriminate MDMA from saline in a two-lever operant paradigm.

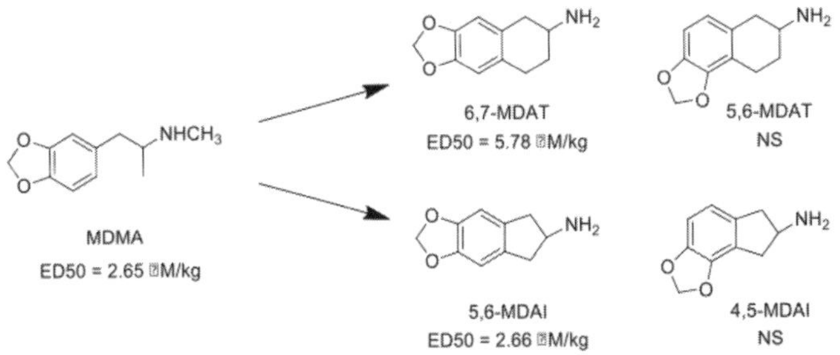

6,7-MDAT
ED50 = 5.78 ⊠M/kg

5,6-MDAT
NS

MDMA
ED50 = 2.65 ⊠M/kg

5,6-MDAI
ED50 = 2.66 ⊠M/kg

4,5-MDAI
NS

We also attempted to determine the relative importance of each of the two oxygen atoms in the methylenedioxy ring of MDA/MDMA (Monte, Marona-Lewicka et al. 1993). That work led to two compounds,

6-APBF and 5-APBF, both of which also subsequently appeared on the research chemicals market. Again, in the figure below, the numbers below each structure are the ED50 values when the compounds were tested in rats trained to discriminate MDMA from saline.

DOM (STP) Hallucinogen	MMA Nonhallucinogen	MMAI 5-HT Releaser	
No substitution	ED50 = 2.74 M/kg	ED50 = 3.77 M/kg	ED50 = 4.06 M/kg

6-APBF	5-APBF	IndanylAMP
ED50 = 1.68 M/kg	ED50 = 1.72 M/kg	ED50 = 0.62 M/kg

Another compound we studied was 5-iodo-2-aminoindan (5-IAI) as a potentially non-neurotoxic analogue of MDMA (Nichols, Johnson et al. 1991). In that case, we had made a radioactive form of it in an attempt to use it as a ligand to label the serotonin reuptake site. 5-IAI also appeared as a research chemical.

With respect to ergolines related to LSD, we synthesised and tested compounds where the N(6) methyl of LSD was replaced by larger alkyl groups. In rats, the N(6)-allyl (allad) proved most potent in a test of LSD-like potency, with the N(6)-ethyl (ethlad) slightly less potent, but more potent than LSD (Hoffman and Nichols, 1985). Both allad and ethlad have now appeared on the research chemical market.

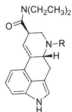

ED50 values from LSD-Trained Rats

R	ED50	Potency relative to LSD*
H	No sub	NA
CH_3 (LSD)	0.046	1.00
CH_2CH_3 (Ethlad)	0.020	2.30
C_3H_7 (ProLad)	0.037	1.24
CH_2CHCH_2 (ALLAD)	0.013	3.54
$CH(CH_3)_2$ iPrLAD	0.10	0.46
C_4H_9 (BuLAD)	0.357	0.13
CH_2CH_2Ph	No sub	NA

*Based on ED50s. Reported values differ and are based on 3 x 3 pt parallel line bioassay.

In another study of LSD-like compounds, we prepared the lysergic acid amides of the three isomers of 2,4-dimethylazetidine: cis, R,R, and S,S dimethyl azetidine (Nichols, Frescas et al. 2002). Both affinity and functional tests at the human 5-HT2A receptor demonstrated that the S,S azetidide was the isomer with pharmacology closest to LSD. That compound also has appeared on the research chemical market as 'LSZ.' We also determined that the diethyl group of LSD interacts with residue Leucine 229, in the loop that connects the top of helix 4 with the top of helix 5 in the 5-HT2A receptor.

$380 \rightarrow 4200$ (11X) $1900 \rightarrow 8700$ (4.6X) $1300 \rightarrow 7900$ (6X)

$68 \rightarrow 2700$ (40X) $2.8 \rightarrow 1435$ (510X)

Finally, we did extensive work on the N-2-methoxybenzyl phenethylamines that became known as NBOMe compounds. Mutagenesis studies of the 5-HT2A receptor indicated that the high potency of these compounds was likely do to a pi-pi interaction between the N-benzyl group of the NBOMe compounds and phenylalanine 339 in the 5-HT2A receptor (Braden, Parrish et al. 2006). The NBOMe compounds have also appeared on the research chemical market, often masquerading on blotters as LSD due to their very high potency. In the figure above, the number on the left is the affinity (in nM) of the compound at the human 5-HT2A receptor, and the number to the right of the arrow is the affinity in the receptor where phenylalanine 339 has been mutated to a leucine residue.

In each case, our molecules were designed to be used as pharmacological tools, to gain a better understanding of how these various molecules interacted with their biological targets. Unfortunately, when we optimised a molecule for biological activity in vitro or in rats, it was often an opportunity for someone to use our published results to market a new research chemical, such as the ones I have talked about above.

Sources:

Braden, M.R., Parrish, J.C., Naylor, J.C., Nichols, D.E. 'Molecular interaction of serotonin 5-HT2A receptor residues Phe339(6.51) and Phe340(6.52) with superpotent N-benzyl phenethylamine agonists.' *Mol Pharmacol.* 2006 70(6):1956–1964.

Hoffman, A.J., Nichols, D.E. 'Synthesis and LSD-like discriminative stimulus properties in a series of N(6)-alkyl norlysergic acid N,N-diethylamide derivatives.' *J Med Chem.* 1985 28(9):1252–1255.

Monte, A.P., Marona-Lewicka, D., Cozzi, N.V, Nichols, D.E. 'Synthesis and pharmacological examination of benzofuran, indan, and tetralin analogues of 3,4-(methylenedioxy) amphetamine.' *J Med Chem.* 1993 36(23):3700–3706.

Nichols, D.E. 'Differences between the mechanism of action of MDMA, MBDB, and the classic hallucinogens. Identification of a new therapeutic class: entactogens.' *J Psychoactive Drugs.* 1986 18(4):305–313.

Nichols, D.E., Brewster, W.K., Johnson, M.P., Oberlender, R., Riggs, R.M. 'Nonneurotoxic tetralin and indan analogues of 3,4- (methylenedioxy)amphetamine (MDA).' *J Med Chem.* 1990 33(2):703–710.

Nichols, D.E., Frescas, S., Marona-Lewicka, D., Kurrasch-Orbaugh, D.M. 'Lysergamides of isomeric 2,4-dimethylazetidines map the binding orientation of the diethylamide moiety in the potent hallucinogenic agent N,N-diethyllysergamide (LSD).' *J Med Chem.* 2002 45(19):4344–4349.

Nichols, D.E., Hoffman, A.J., Oberlender, R.A., Jacob III, P., Shulgin, A.T. 'Derivatives of 1-(1,3-benzodioxol-5-yl)-2-butanamine: representatives of a novel therapeutic class.' *J Med Chem.* 1986 29(10): 2009–2015, 1986.

Nichols, D.E., Johnson, M.P., Oberlender, R. '5-Iodo-2-aminoindan, a non-neurotoxic analogue of p-iodoamphetamine.' *Pharmacol Biochem Behav.* 1991 38(1):135–139.

CASE REPORT OF A HIGH FREQUENCY, NON-CLINICAL HALLUCINOGEN USER

JENNIFER LYKE AND JULIA KUTI

Users report a wide range of benefits from hallucinogenic drug use.[1] In particular, psilocybin has been investigated recently for its role in inducing mystical experiences, and it has been shown that these experiences continue to have effects up to three years after the initial experience.[2]

Among other effects, psilocybin appears to bias perception and mood positively[3] and to alter personality in the direction of increased openness,[4] and in fact psychedelic drug users differ significantly from users of other drugs in spiritual values and empathy.[5] In addition, the peak experiences of psilocybin users that occur with psilocybin use are unique.[6]

Case studies play an important role in highlighting particular experiences in a population of interest. To date, case studies have investigated psilocybin as a treatment for Obsessive-Compulsive Disorder[7] and Body Dysmorphic Disorder.[8] Another case report documented an incident of Hallucinogen Persisting Perceptual Disorder related to psilocybin use,[9] but no research has yet investigated unique individual cases of hallucinogen use in the non-clinical population.

This research reports on the investigation of a particular non-clinical case, which is notable due to the frequency and duration of psilocybin use. Mark (not his real name) reported that he used a large amount of psilocybin (between one and ten grams) almost daily for approximately ten months with no negative consequences. In addition, he reported that he experienced substantive changes in the content and quality of his awareness. Hopefully, describing this case will be useful to future investigations of effects of high frequency psilocybin use in naturalistic settings.

METHOD

Mark was a 24-year old, Caucasian male, working full time as a driver making deliveries for a local company, who was suggested by one of his friends as a guest speaker for an undergraduate class addressing the topic of hallucinogens and their effects on consciousness. He agreed to be interviewed for the class and signed a consent form to be used as the subject of a case study. Mark participated in two interviews, approximately one hour each, intended to investigate the possible effects of his extended psilocybin use on his awareness. During those interviews and in response to subsequent follow-up questions, Mark described his experiences with hallucinogenic drugs and his view of reality, which he perceived to be quite different from ordinary people's views.

RESULTS

Mark reported that he had taken psilocybin mushrooms almost daily for approximately ten months, with one or two weeks of abstinence during that time. He estimated his usual dose on weekdays was between one and three grams, whereas his usual dose on weekends was five to ten grams. He reported that the highest dose he ever consumed was approximately twenty grams. He did not believe he had developed a tolerance to psilocybin during the course of his high-frequency use. He also did not believe that high doses affected him differently than lower doses, apart from his perception that higher doses extended the effect of the drug.

Mark had a full-time job driving for a local company. He graduated from high school and had one year of college. He was not currently in a romantic relationship. He reported first smoking marijuana when he was 17, and that he never enjoyed alcohol. He reported that he first took psilocybin when he was 19, but had a particularly meaningful experience on psilocybin when he was 23, after which he decided to take psilocybin regularly for an undetermined period of time. Mark reported using alcohol occasionally but that he did not use other substances such as opioids, stimulants, or dissociative drugs. Mark denied any relationship problems or problems related to his work or physical health due to his drug use. He reported that he never sought mental health treatment, never had legal problems due to his drug use, and was never in a rehabilitation programme for substance abuse.

Mark reported he chose to end his regular psilocybin use after ten months essentially as another phase of the 'experiment'. He stated that he wanted to determine whether he would have cravings and how his awareness might change during abstinence from psilocybin. After approximately five months of abstinence, Mark reported he had no signs of withdrawal, but that he would continue to take psilocybin at his previous rate if he had access to it. He cited the allure of the insights experienced under the influence of psilocybin as the reason he would continue to take it regularly. He also indicated that he believed his perspective had been permanently altered in a profound and positive way.

TRANSCENDENT CONSCIOUSNESS

Mark described his psilocybin-induced perspective as qualitatively different than ordinary awareness in important ways. For example, he interpreted his experience as involving greater access to the unconscious and increased intuition compared to ordinary consciousness. He described ordinary awareness as excessively limited when viewed from the psilocybin-induced state:

It's like a hamster running on a wheel, and then when you introduce psilocybin, the hamster starts looking around and says, 'I don't need to run on this wheel anymore. There's a lot of room to move around in here. What the f--- am I doing?' And you start to de-prioritize, organize, prioritize everything that you've ever been and everything that you've ever experienced.

Similarly, he described a sense of understanding of fundamental truths induced by psilocybin: 'Psilocybin is a rebirth, a re-understanding of who you should be and how you should live—how you should treat others.' Other examples of principles Mark understood as truths revealed by psilocybin included the oneness of all things and the illusions created by the egocentric state of ordinary awareness: 'The ego makes you fear things. There's nothing to fear. Death isn't real.'

Mark described a uniquely noetic quality to his awareness, which he attributed directly to psilocybin: 'It's like the lazy man's discovery. You take a large dose and they're giving you the answers. It's the cheat sheet that wasn't given out in class.' He also emphasised the uniqueness of the insights he experienced, which he believed could only be achieved with psilocybin: 'On these you experience so much. It's an incredible lucidity of understanding or knowing. And if you're not on them and you never experienced them, *you don't f---ing know.*' He summarised the experience as fundamentally 'profound' and expressed the ineffability that is characteristic of mystical experiences: 'Language is a lie... The words I've been using are a complete injustice to what the experience is.'

Finally, Mark repeatedly reiterated that psilocybin was both necessary and sufficient to achieve the insights he felt he had received and suggested that the alternative reality induced by psilocybin facilitates one's ability to 'unlock the cage' of conditioning, the ultimate purpose of which is to realise 'life is about caring for one another and this organism that we live on.' According to Mark, psilocybin teaches these lessons by communicating the realisation that '[i]t's all about you. It's all about what's going on between your ears. It has nothing to do with anything else... [Psilocybin is] meant for the finding and education of yourself—*the* Self.'

GRANDIOSITY AND DELUSIONS

During the interviews, Mark repeatedly expressed a sense that he understood reality differently than other people and implied that ordinary understanding of reality was inferior to his own. He seemed either unaware or unconcerned that his presentation appeared dismissive of other perspectives. He viewed his specialness as deriving directly from the insights he gained from psilocybin, but he discounted suggestions that his unique perspective might create a barrier for relationships between himself and others with more ordinary frames of consciousness. He denied feeling lonely due to his unique state.

In addition, Mark mentioned several ideas that he viewed as factual, which appear delusional from the perspective of ordinary awareness. For example, Mark said that he had communicated telepathically with a cat and that he could drive with his eyes closed for miles while on psilocybin. He also believed he could 'astral travel' while under the influence of psilocybin and alluded to several beliefs implying conspiracies among the cultural elite to control the minds and lives of the unsuspecting public. For example, he said that television 'exists to put you in a false reality,' which, of course, is true. However, the implicit meaning of his statement appeared to include the sense that some elements of the dominant social structure have purposefully designed television in this way in order to gain power or resources from it, which, of course, is also true. This aspect of the conversation served as a useful example of a legitimate statement that could be interpreted as Mark's astute perception of the sociopolitical principles underlying cultural realities or as Mark's tendency toward paranoia infusing his perception of a simple fact.

Mark also expressed unique beliefs about the significance of psilocybin mushrooms in human history, including that all plant life on Earth is due to mushrooms and all religion stems from early human hallucinogenic experiences. He also suggested major cultural myths and symbols, such as the myth of the Phoenix, Easter egg hunts, and the Arthurian legend of the sword in the stone, all originated specifically as symbolic representations of historical human experience with mushrooms. Mark explicitly expressed an inflexibility regarding these beliefs and an unwillingness to consider any ambiguity about these interpretations.

DISCUSSION

The most notable aspect of Mark's experience was the frequency and duration with which he reported having used psilocybin. While there are no reports of average frequency of psilocybin use in the medical or psychological literature, almost daily use for approximately ten months is likely to be far beyond the frequency and duration of ordinary psilocybin users. For this reason, Mark's case is notable as a naturalistic example of the effects of high frequency use over an extended period of time. Although there is no independent evidence supporting Mark's assertions regarding his psilocybin use, and therefore his reports may be exaggerated or inaccurate, there is likewise no evidence contradicting his report. Future research investigating rates of high frequency hallucinogen use would be helpful in determining the likelihood that Mark's report is accurate.

Accordingly, Mark's description of his awareness after several months of daily psilocybin use raises several important points. First, it is clear that his subjective experience involved a sense of intuitive realisation of deep, transcendent truths he believed were facilitated by his psilocybin use. Indeed, this conclusion is consistent with controlled studies of psilocybin's ability to induce mystical experiences.[10-11] Mark's sense that his awareness was permanently altered is also consistent with research indicating that even single episodes of psilocybin use can have long-lasting effects.[4, 10] Mark's descriptions of his insights substantively match reports of participants in other studies.[1, 12]

In addition, it is notable that Mark reported no social, occupational, legal, financial, or health problems secondary to his psilocybin use.

However, it is important to acknowledge there is no independent verification of any information Mark reported. Therefore, it is possible that either Mark's report of problems is understated, that his perception of his functioning differs from the perceptions of others in his life, or that his report regarding his frequency or duration of use is inaccurate. In particular, Mark clearly stated that he did not experience symptoms of substance dependence, such as cravings or withdrawal symptoms, after stopping his daily use, but it is unclear to what extent psychological dependence and/or tolerance may have played a role in the frequency or amount of his use over an extended period of time. There is very little discussion of the role of spiritual experiences in motivating drug use, especially hallucinogens, but this case may be an example of compulsive hallucinogen use driven by the allure of transcendent awareness.

Some of Mark's beliefs are consistent with those of a subculture of hallucinogen proponents. Therefore, it is difficult to determine to what extent Mark's perspective was directly induced by psilocybin versus to what extent he adopted the perspective of the subculture to which he belonged. For example, McKenna[13] has proposed that psilocybin mushrooms played a central role in human spiritual and cultural evolution, and McKenna is a well-known figure among hallucinogen users. However, ideas about the centrality of psilocybin mushrooms in human history could also arise as a projection of the user's assessment of the importance of his own experience.

In particular, the notion that psilocybin mushrooms are integrally related to the history of human spiritual development may stem, at least partially, from the unique noetic sense induced by psilocybin. Perspectives that appear delusional to those in ordinary reality may reflect the dramatically different quality of the psilocybin-induced state. For example, telepathy and astral projection may represent important symbolic aspects of the experience, namely special abilities that are supernatural relative to ordinary awareness. Similarly, belief in large-scale conspiracies may symbolically represent the misleading values propagated by the dominant sociopolitical structure that contribute to the sense of disconnection and alienation of those in ordinary awareness. In other words, it may be that seemingly delusional or grandiose aspects of the drug-induced experience can be interpreted as vividly manifested aspects of ordinary unconscious contents.

Finally, Mark's case may not be as unique as it appears. It is possible that there are other cases of high frequency psilocybin use that go undetected by the health care or legal systems because, if Mark is correct, such patterns of use do not necessarily cause functional difficulties. Future research should address this issue by attempting to identify similar cases in the general population, and by estimating the average frequency of use among psilocybin users. In addition, it would be helpful to establish basic demographic statistics (average age, level of education, race/ethnicity) of psilocybin users since there is no way at this time to determine to what extent Mark's characteristics are typical of psilocybin users generally.

Recent research has identified young adulthood as a time of unique risk of experimentation with consciousness-altering substances.[15] Although Mark is almost certainly an outlier, his case may characterise important elements of young people's experience, especially those seeking a particular type of transcendent knowledge which is not readily available in modern culture. Future researchers investigating extreme uses of psilocybin should be careful to consider the needs such patterns of use meet, as well as the risks they may present to developing adults.

References:

1. Carhart-Harris, R.L., Nutt, D.J. 'User perceptions of the benefits and harms of hallucinogenic drug use: a web-based questionnaire study'. *J Subst Use.* 2010 15(4):283–300.

2. Griffiths, R., Richards, W., McCann, U., Jesse, R. 'Psilocybin can occasion mystical-type experiences having substantial and sustained personal meaning and spiritual significance'. In *Psychedelic medicine: new evidence for hallucinogenic substances as treatments.* Vol 2. Winkelman, M.J. (ed). Westport, CT: Praeger Publishers/Greenwood Publishing Group. 2006.

3. Kometer, M., Schmidt, A., Bachmann, R., Studerus, E., Seifritz, E., Vollenweider, F.X. 'Psilocybin biases facial recognition, goal-directed behavior, and mood state toward positive relative to negative emotions through different serotonergic subreceptors'. *Biol Psychiatry.* 2012 72:898–906.

4. MacLean, K.A., Johnson, M.W., Griffiths, R.R. 'Mystical experiences occasioned by the hallucinogen psilocybin lead to increases in the personality domain of openness'. *J Psychopharmacol.* 2011 25(11):1453–1461.

5. Lerner, M., Lyvers, M. 'Values and beliefs of psychedelic drug users: a cross-cultural study'. *J Psychoactive Drugs.* 2006 38(2):143–147.

6. Cummins, C., Lyke, J. 'Peak experiences of psilocybin users and non-users'. *J Psychoactive Drugs.* 2013 45(2):189–194.

7. Moreno, F.A., Delgado, P.L. 'Hallucinogen-induced relief of obsessions and compulsions'. *Am J Psychiatry.* 1997 154(7):1037.

8. Hanes, K.R. 'Serotonin, psilocybin, and Body Dysmorphic Disorder: a case report'. *J Clin Psychopharmacol.* 1996 16(2):188–189.

9. Espiard, M., Lecardeur, L., Abadie, P., Halbecqu, I., Dollfus, S. 'Hallucinogen persisting perception disorder after psilocybin consumption: a case study'. *Eur Psychiatry.* 2005 20:458–460.

10. Griffiths, R.R., Richards, W.A., Johnson, M.W., McCann, U.D., Jesse, R. 'Mystical-type experiences occasioned by psilocybin mediate the attribution of personal meaning and spiritual significance 14 months later'. *J Psychopharmacol.* 2008 22(6):621–632.

11. Pahnke, W.N. 'Drugs and mysticism'. *IJP.* 1966 8:295–314.

12. Carhart-Harris, R.L., Nutt, D.J. 'Experienced drug users assess the relative harms and benefits of drugs: a web-based survey'. *J Psychoactive Drugs.* 2013 45(4):322–328.

13. McKenna, T. *Food of the Gods: the search for the original tree of knowledge.* New York: Bantam Books. 1992.

14. Stone, A.L., Becker, L.G., Huber, A.M., Catalano, R.F. 'Review of risk and protective factors of substance use and problem use in emerging adulthood'. *Addict Behav.* 2012 37:747–775.

SAVING AND ARCHIVING THE WORLD LITERATURE ON PSYCHEDELIC DRUGS:

WHAT GOOGLE'S NGRAM VIEWER TELLS US

MICHAEL MONTAGNE

In 1970, four book collectors merged their private libraries to create the Fitz Hugh Ludlow Memorial Library, the first organised, non-academic based attempt at saving and archiving literature on psychoactive drugs.[1] This was followed closely in the early 1970s by the Schaffer Library of Drug Policy and the Drug Information Service Center at the University of Minnesota's College of Pharmacy, both of which catalogued many historical and contemporary works on psychedelic drugs. With the tragically chilling effect of the conservative 1980s, some of these libraries closed or went silent. A resurgence of interest in psychedelic drugs in the 1990s, combined with the emerging Internet, led to the creation of new archives with easily accessed online databases including Erowid (1995), The Lycaeum (1996), and Purdue University's Psychoactive Substances Research Collection (2006). Specialty collections on individual drugs have also been created such as 'Shroomery' which focuses on psychoactive mushrooms.

In 2003, the Ludlow Library, which had been in storage while searching for a new home for decades, became part of the Ludlow Santo Domingo Library in Geneva, Switzerland, and after the death of its owner, Julio Mario Santo Domingo, Jr. in 2009, that collection was loaned by the family to Harvard University.[2] But is one massive collection of drug literature in a single physical location, or meagerly funded information websites, enough to save this literature for future generations of drug users and researchers? And outside of books by well-known publishers, is there a need to save and archive historical ephemera, documents related to important events, self-published works, and private libraries?

At the Breaking Convention 3 conference held in Greenwich, UK, in July 2015, I presented on the application of Google's Ngram Analytic Tool to the world literature on psychedelic drugs. My research showed that the Ngram Viewer appears to be a functional tool for performing searches on the usage popularity of words and phrases related to psychedelic drugs over the past century. It also showed how little of the known body of psychedelic drug literature is being mega-archived and recognised by search engines and high-throughput analyses. The full presentation can be viewed at Breaking Convention videos on Vimeo (https://vimeo.com/ecologycosmos).

After my presentation and during the remainder of the conference, participants approached me to discuss the need to save all types of literature and materials (film, art, etc.) on psychedelic drugs. As I stood before the booksellers' tables at the conference, I wondered how many of those books and magazines would be saved and made available 50 years from now. The world of information changes quickly, drastically, ephemerally, and much has already been lost forever.

The utility of the Ngram Viewer, while the focus of my presentation, will be discussed herein as a foundation to formulate an argument for the need to save and archive literature and materials on psychedelic drugs. The results of the application of the Ngram Viewer to the world literature on psychedelic drugs are presented first to portray its utility as a research tool. These results then identify a more urgent need to collectively save and archive these materials.

GOOGLE'S NGRAM VIEWER ANALYTIC TOOL

The research utility of the Ngram Viewer analytic tool applied to drug literature was examined in a previous study by this author.[3] It is a useful tool for discovering the popularity of drug words over the past four centuries. Problems using the Viewer occurred with the choice of words or phrases, language choice, time frames under study, and the meaning of results obtained. The following was described in that study:[3]

> Google Inc. has archived over 15 million books which represent approximately 12% of all published books from 1500 to 2008.[4] These books were scanned and digitized from copies residing in approximately 40 participating libraries using optical character recognition (OCR), a technology that identifies the image of a word in the scanning process and then stores it digitally. The accuracy of this technology depends on the software's ability to recognize letters in the word thus identifying the word for proper digital storage for later recall and use. This differs from direct replication of text such as photocopying or scanning it as a 'picture' for a pdf file (portable document format by Adobe Reader®).
>
> A research group has taken a corpus (body) of this digitized library amounting to approximately 8.1 million book and created a database for computational analysis of specific words and phrases that are in these scanned books.[5-7] The analytic tool developed for searching the Google Books database is called Ngram Viewer and Version 1 was released for use on December 16, 2010. The primary purpose of this tool is to perform 'culturomics' research, 'the application of high-throughput data collection and analysis to the study of human culture.'[6]

The Google Books Ngram Viewer is designed for inquiries into the presence or usage of words and phrases in the scanned book database. An n-gram is a sequence of 1-grams, which are strings of text characters uninterrupted by a space; they are words, acronyms, numbers, and even typographical errors.[6] The corpus limits the 1-grams to a maximum number of five (ex., five separate words or comprising a phrase), and the n-gram must occur at least 40 times in the corpus. The most recent version (2.0) of this database was released in July 2012 and represents scanned books published through 2008.[5] In Version 2.0 the n-grams are grouped alphabetically (languages with non-Latin scripts were transliterated). A summary of how the corpus was constructed can be found at http://books.google.com/ngrams/info. This compilation is licensed under a Creative Commons Attribution 3.0 Unported License.

To use the Viewer, one to five words, or a phrase of not more than five words, are entered into the n-gram box. The range of years to be reviewed and language corpus are selected, along with choice of smoothing function. The smoothing function refers to viewing the data as a moving average. The smoothing number represents the number of years on either side of the given year that are included in calculating the average. A smoothing of four means that the raw count for a given year, for instance 1950, is added to the raw counts for the four years on either side of the given year, and then the total raw count is divided by the number of years, in this case by nine (1946–1954). The larger the smoothing number, the more years on either side of a given year are used in averaging, and the flatter the peaks on the curve. No smoothing means no averages, only raw data are graphed. While no rule or suggestion has been provided to date in studies on the Ngram Viewer, the assessment performed in this study suggests that a smoothing number between three and five allows for some control over variation in number of books published in a given year balanced with an ability to identify important peaks of activity or usage of the key word or phrase.

The search is initiated with the user determined parameters of words/phrases, range of years, and smoothing function, and the results are displayed graphically with curves for each search word or phrase on a chart by year. The x-axis has coordinates in years and the y-axis has coordinates in percentages of scanned books that contain the ngram.

Below the chart, categories of years in the given range by word/phrase are supplied. These provide a link to the listing of scanned books in the given year range.

A number of issues and problems have been identified by users of the Ngram Viewer.[8-10] The major issue is the use of the OCR scanning technology and its misinterpretation of letters and words in the digitisation process. One example is the medial 's' when the letter 'f' is used in place of 's' in older texts.[9] The Viewer's results show popularity of usage of words and phrases, but they don't explain why they were popular. Meanings of words and phrases can change over time, and this problem is not directly identifiable in the results.[10] The choice of dates and smoothing function can skew results. Work on the Ngram Viewer Version 1 produced a much improved Version 2. ORC scanning technology and metadata extraction techniques have been improved leading to higher quality digitisation of the books. N-grams spanning sentence boundaries have been omitted, and those spanning page boundaries in the text have been included. Statistical models have been developed and implemented to produce syntactic (rules and accepted structures of syntax or grammar) annotations that handle historical text more robustly.'[5]

APPLICATION TO WORLD LITERATURE ON PSYCHEDELIC DRUGS

Searches on general drug words ('psychedelic', 'hallucinogen', and 'entheogen') produced somewhat different results, especially by language. Results from the search words 'psychedelic', 'hallucinogen', and 'entheogen' in the English language for the time period 1950–2005 are presented in FIGURE 1. The y-axis coordinates, originally in percentages of scanned books that contained the ngram, have been converted to the approximate number of books that contained the search word.

The words 'psychedelic' and 'hallucinogen' entered the literature in the 1950s. The word 'psychedelic' quickly peaked in 1971 and then declined until an upturn in popularity began around 1990. The 1971 peak

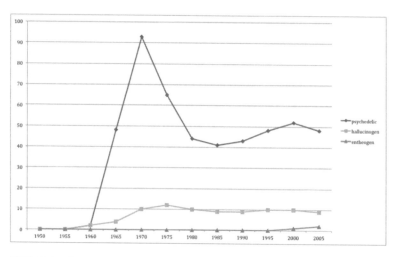

FIGURE 1: Results from search words: psychedelic, hallucinogen, entheogen (English corpus, 1950–2005).

represented just over 90 books with that word. 'Hallucinogen' began to increase in popularity in the late 1960s, and has remained consistent with no other increases or peaks. Entheogen had very limited popularity in the literature, amounting to just two books in 2005. Part of the 'psychedelic' peak around 1970 included uses of the word not directly connected to drugs, but instead the larger cultural use of the term to represent art, music, and other aspects of society during that time.

When the search was limited to English literature published only in America, the results did not change much at all from those in FIGURE 1. When the search was limited to English literature published only in Great Britain, the curve for 'psychedelic' changed noticeably with a large increase in popularity beginning in 1990 and still increasing; the 1971 peak was narrower. When the search was limited to English fiction, the second growth of popularity in the 1990s was still evident, though the beginning of this later increase began in 1985.

From searching other languages, the word 'psychedelic' was the more popular term in English, French, and Italian literature, while

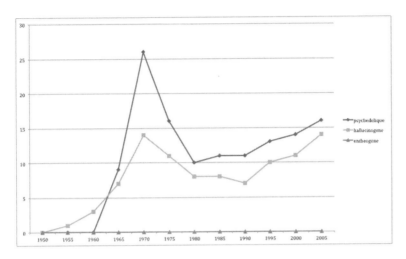

FIGURE 2: Results from search words; psychédélique, hallucinogène, enthéogène (French corpus, 1950–2005).

'hallucinogen' was more popular in German, Spanish, and Russian literature. Use of these search words spelled out in English in other language corpi led to erroneous results. When the three search words were spelled in English and the French literature corpus was searched, 'psychedelic' was the only word that returned results with a peak in 1970 similar to, but shorter than, the other previous examples. Searches using language-specific translated versions of those three terms were necessary to produce more precise results.

When the French spelling of the search words 'psychédélique', 'hallucinogène', and 'enthéogène' were used for the period 1950–2005 in searching the French literature corpus, the curve (FIGURE 2) was similar to that for English (FIGURE 1), but 'hallucinogène' showed a smaller peak in 1970, increased in 1977 to pass the popularity of 'psychédélique', and then 'psychédélique' became more popular in 2003. Was 'hallucinogène' the favoured word in French literature for that 25 year period? This curve for 'hallucinogène' was not similar to that found in the English language searches.

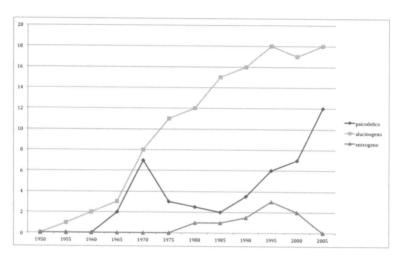

FIGURE 3: Results from search words: psicodélico, alucinógeno, enteógeno (Spanish corpus, 1950–2005).

Searches in the Spanish, German, Italian, and Russian languages, using the spellings of the three search words in those languages, returned a range of different results, though for the most part the popularity of the words 'psychedelic' and 'hallucinogen' increased throughout the later part of the 20th century and into the 21st century. In the Spanish literature (1950–2005), 'psicodélico', 'alucinógeno', and 'enteógeno' all returned results (FIGURE 3), the first language in which the word 'entheogen' showed any level of cultural popularity in any of the corpi examined in this study. 'Alucinógeno' was the most popular term throughout the timeframe of study, consistently increasing in popularity with no real separate peak, averaging approximately 17 books per year since 1990. 'Psicodélico' showed the typical peak in 1970, followed by a decline and then a continued increase from 1990 to today. 'Enteógeno' showed popularity in this language, though less than the other two terms, with peak activity in the 1990s and declining since then.

'Halluzinogen' was more popular than 'psychedelisch' in the German literature (1950–2005) with a peak in 1972 plus additional

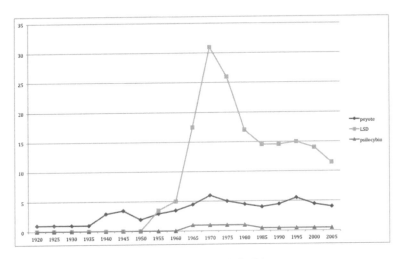

FIGURE 4: Results from search words: peyote, LSD, psilocybin (English corpus, 1920–2005).

peaks in the early 1990s and early 2000s. In the Italian literature (1950-2005), 'allucinogeno' and 'psichedelico' were relatively equal in popularity from peaks in 1969 and 1971 respectively, followed with an even larger peak for both in 1998. In Russian (1950–2005), 'психоделика' (psychedelic) and 'галлюциноген' (hallucinogen) became popular later than in the US and Western European countries. The search word 'галлюциноген' (hallucinogen) first appeared in 1964, and its popularity has been increasing since then. The search word 'психоделика' (psychedelic) first appeared in 1985, peaked in 1995, then declined slightly, before increasing in popularity.

Employing search words that are specific drug names ('peyote', 'LSD', 'psilocybin') produced even more precise results, such as the example in English over the time period 1920–2005 (FIGURE 4). These same search words ('peyote', 'LSD', 'psilocybin'), in the spelling of the language corpus being searched, revealed interesting results in French, Spanish, Italian, German, and Russian over the same time period. In all languages, except Spanish, 'LSD' was consistently the most popular term, usually with a peak around 1970, the exception being in Italian when the word first reached peak popularity in 1958. In all languages, except English, 'LSD' has been increasing in popularity from the 1990s onward. The French, German and Russian curves for 'LSD' were similar to the one in English. 'LSD' occurred in the Russian language before 1940 which must be due to the use of that three-letter acronym for something other than the drug.

The word 'peyote' was popular in the Spanish language corpus exceeding 'LSD' in popularity from 1978 to 2005, with a number of peaks in the late 1920s, 1940, early 1970s, and early 2000s. The popularity of the word 'peyote' matched that of 'LSD' in Spanish. 'Peyote' in the other languages presented a curve similar to the one for it in English, with a peak in 1970 in the French corpus, and a minor degree of popularity in Italian, German, and Russian. The word 'psilocybin' had not been popular at any time in Spanish or Russian, and only briefly in the 1960s in French (Roger Heim's work), German, and Italian. Another peak in popularity in the Italian corpus occurred in the late 1990s and early 2000s.

The search words 'caapi', 'yage', 'yaje', and 'ayahuasca' (English corpus, 1900–2005) returned results that showed a general popularity that was greatest in the 1970s. The word 'caapi' had popularity peaks in 1905–10, the 1920s, 1940s, and 1970s. The search word 'yage' peaked in the late 1970s and early 1980s and again in the 1990s. It also was noted that some literature items in the corpus identified the word 'v'yage' (voyage) as 'yage' in the search process, presenting a problem in the interpretation of its curve. The word 'yaje' peaked also in the 1970s with another peak in the 2000s. The word 'ayahuasca' also peaked in the 1970s and has become the most popular word of the four from about 1983 onwards. The search words 'Iboga', 'ibogaine', 'Salvia divinorum', and 'salvinorin A' (English corpus, 1950-2005) showed little popularity compared to other drugs, with 'ibogaine' the most popular word with a peak in the 1960s and greater popularity from 1995 to 2005. 'Salvia divinorum' and 'salvinorin A' have shown increased popularity since 2000.

The Viewer and OCR technology will continue to improve, and that will enhance the tool's ability to correctly identify words and retrieve more accurate data for graphic display. There still are potential problems in using the Viewer, in terms of choice of words, time frames, and the meaning of results obtained. This analytic tool can supplement other research methods to study drugs on the Internet (3). The application of high-throughput data collection and analysis to the study of human culture, called 'culturomics,' should be useful in studies on the historical epidemiology of drug use, mass media representations of psychedelic drugs and their use, and adoption and regulation of psychedelic drug technologies.

SAVING CULTURAL LITERATURE ON PSYCHEDELIC DRUGS

This evaluative study of the Ngram Viewer found that it has utility as a research tool and a measure of the popularity of specific words related to psychedelic drugs. Keeping in mind that Google has archived only 12% of published books from 1500 to 2005, and only about 7% are available for word searches using the Viewer, the results presented herein are obviously limited. It was noticeable however that the number of books and related print material on psychedelic drugs archived by Google is small in comparison to other drugs such as opium, alcohol, cannabis/marijuana, and others, for which hundreds of books per year have already been archived in the Google database. The closest number in this study was almost 90 books in English with the word 'psychedelic' during the height of its popularity in 1970.

Anthologies and other print compilations of drug literature in the 1960s and 1970s educated a generation of drug users. Introduction to original sources occurred through their identification in these books and early collections. Knowledgeable users and researchers studied early accounts of psychedelic drug experiences to learn, understand, and enhance their own investigations and experiences. Contemporary bibliographies and other comprehensive compilations are limited, except perhaps for LSD (which tend to cover only the medical-scientific literature). There is a great need to develop and publish in open source literature.

There is a fragility to online and even print archives that can be closed or disassembled for various reasons. As of now, few books on psychedelic drugs are being broadly archived. These archives are vulnerable. Archiving done by most academic libraries and other groups typically misses a lot of this literature, such as: self-published works; works from little know publishers or the 'underground' press (which for the most part is not underground anymore, given the Internet); ephemera, unique, and one-of-a-kind items; works lost due to a lack of collecting with the intent to save; and works not saved due to a lack of interest in or even prohibition from including these topics by most libraries.

Knowledgeable psychedelic drug users should have a personal responsibility to document their experiences, learn from those of other users (the literature on experiences), and to collect, save, and archive this literature for future generations.

References:

1. Dailey Rare Books. The Fitz Hugh Ludlow Memorial Library. Available from: http://daileyrarebooks.com/ludlow.htm

2. Houghton Library. Harvard University. The Julio Mario Santo Domingo collection. Available from: http://hcl.harvard.edu/libraries/houghton/collections/modern/santo_domingo.cfm

3. Montagne, M., Morgan, M. 'Drugs on the Internet, part IV: Google's Ngram viewer analytic tool applied to drug literature'. *Substance Use & Misuse*. 2013 48:415-19.

4. Wikipedia. Google Ngram Viewer. September 29 2012. Available from: http://en.wikipedia.org/wiki/Google_Ngram_Viewer

5. Lin, Y., Michel, J-B., Aiden, E.L., Orwant, J., Brockman, W., Petrov, S. 'Syntactic annotations for the Google books Ngram corpus'. Proceed 50th Ann Meet Assoc Comput Ling. 2012:169-74. Available from: http://aclweb.org/anthology-new/P/P12/P12-3029.pdf

6. Michel, J-B., Shen, Y.K., Aiden, A.P., Veres, A., Gray, M.K., The Google Book Team, et al. 'Quantitative analysis of culture using millions of digitized books'. *Science*. 2011 331:176-82.

7. Orwant, J. Google Research Blog [Internet]. Ngram viewer 2.0. October 18 2012. Available from: http://googleresearch.blogspot.com/

8. Russell, M. 'Google database tracks popularity of 500B words'. newser. December 17 2010. Available from: http://www.newser.com/story/107766/google-database-tracks-popularity-of-500b-words.html

9. Sullivan, D. 'When OCR goes bad: Google's Ngram viewer and the F-word'. Search Engine Land. December 19 2010. Available from: http://searchengineland.com/when-ocr-goes-badgoogles-ngram-viewer-the-f-word-59181

10. Whitney, L. 'Google's Ngram viewer: a time machine for wordplay'. c/net. December 17 2010. Available from: http://news.cnet.com/8301-1023_3-20025979-93.html

TRANSGRESSION AND ECONOMY DURING DRUG REFORM

JONATHAN NEWMAN

Ongoing legal reforms increase the possibilities of legitimate cannabis economies, yet what sort of cannabis markets do we want? The question extends beyond cannabis to other drugs under control too. Legal reforms governing the production, processing and circulation of cannabis (or specific cannabinoids), favour some forms of economy over others. The current journey towards legitimation sees drugs (re) framed as relief from a range of ills, and the technological expansion of products. These are fertile grounds to advance commoditised medicated lifestyles.

This paper arose as an off-shoot from my ethnographic research into the Medical Cannabis Bike Tour (MCBT), which I have been studying since 2013. The charity bike ride raises money for Dr Manuel Guzman's research group, at Complutense University of Madrid, who are investigating whether cannabinoids can be used in conjunction with existing treatments for gliomas (a type of brain tumour).

The cycle ride is run and sponsored by the cannabis industry— the seed breeders, fertilizers and hydroponics companies, rolling papers manufacturers, and cannabis media. It is through their efforts that you have your cannabis. Although they don't produce cannabis (which mostly remains illegal) they do provide the infrastructure for the cannabis economy. All legal economies integrate with illegal economies. It's not just drugs. There are flows of goods, finance and services through the legislative lines of transgression.

Despite operating legally, there is something not quite clean about the cannabis trade—they struggle to be legitimate but 'morality, ambivalence and uncertainty hangs over the cannabis user' (p.147).[1] In Mary Douglas's words, they are 'dirt'—'matter out of place'.[2] One Dutch trader told me that he does not tell the parents of his daughter's school friends that he works in the industry—even though his job is 100% legal under Dutch law. The former Secretary General of Ghana told me at a drug conference: 'The people who smoke this are dirty. We call the stuff weed'. On the bike tour we stop for lunch in a car park by a river in rural Holland, but are moved on almost immediately because of the cannabis users. We are not welcome, we are outsiders.

Much consumption and production in Europe happens outside of state legal sanction with an estimated 22 million consumers (10% from the UK).[3] The struggle for legitimacy takes place while the goods of legal traders in the cannabis trade are entering a criminal economy. Cannabis trading has a modern history of illegality and has cultured meanings of use and trade that straddle categories of unacceptability and danger. Yet categorisation is dependent upon position. We differentiate and distinguish legitimacy according to our own individual and collective histories. Categories of transgression can change again or switch back—sometimes very quickly.

For Roitman, questions about legitimacy need to be addressed by understanding 'the economy as a political terrain' (p.6).[4] Illegal sectors operate within legal sectors, and there is substantial integration—at times they can be at the heart of productive activity. In those unofficial economies, 'you can be in the margins and in the norm' (p.21).[4] Roitman's insights remind us that the boom in cannabis medicines has come out of an illegal sector that considered itself legitimate.

The cannabis industry, by incorporating modern technological horticulture, including selective breeding and genetic modification, has innovated new strains, growing techniques and processing methods. Together with activists operating a cottage industry of self-appointed providers of cannabis treatments (some who see themselves as healers), this productive activity has brought us sufficient anecdotal evidence to steer medical research and contribute towards knowledge on producing cannabinoid concentrates. Scientific researchers are not completely disengaged from the anecdotal evidence of cottage industries, and vice versa.

THE ECONOMIC TERRAIN BUILDING REFORM

Money to be made through transgression fits into existing cultural economies. Research has found that localised drug traffickers 'mastered the art of transgression and discovered the significance of an economy of consumption'.[5] Reform re-orders the points of transgression, simultaneously widening the consumer opportunities in line with an existing ethos of consumption. It's business as usual, but under reform the production of wealth is sanctioned by the (self-sanctioning) state. As such, reform offers entrepreneurs in the cannabis sector the potential of greater trade and profits as well as a more direct route to accumulate and circulate capital.

Individual profiteering is insufficient in itself for reform. For Parry and Bloch,[6] perceived benefits to the collective whole are positively associated with the central moral values of a social group, whereas individual profit is only allowed within certain limits. Or, as a veteran on the bike tour said more succinctly, 'If you don't give something back to society they come and get you'. Reform needs to augment the collective whole by mobilising (within a particular form of economy) models of medicine, taxation, and the reduction of law and order costs.

Hugh-Jones[7] argues that we cannot understand drug taking by indigenous groups in the Amazon using our own social and cosmological ordering; the reverse also applies. We need to understand our own cultural economy to understand the legitimisation of drug use. We live in times of neo-liberal drives that defer governmental responsibilities to private enterprise chasing profits. This ideological movement is also accompanied by economic production that promotes and fulfils mass commodity consumption, such that 'the economy produces goods and goods are good so more goods must be better' (p.24).[8] Under more relaxed laws, 'multi-nationals and small time entrepreneurs see the opportunity of profits to be gained' (p.128).[9]

Joop Oomen, co-founder of ENCOD, told me about the unexpected direction of reform. After years of activism, he has seen many of the non-profit Cannabis Social Clubs turn into profit making organisations with private investors. In the US, some of same people who were campaigning for reform are now legal commercial growers who, to secure their own profits, lobby Washington to prevent private growing.

Stock market and venture capital have entered the US cannabis business. Robert Farrell is the marketing strategist for CannLabs, a stock market listed company in Denver, Colorado, that does cannabis testing and helps with state and industry drafting of new regulations. Robert previously worked leading marketing strategies for Royal Bank of Scotland. He doesn't smoke—he's just not that kind of person—he's there to do a job, making money for himself and the company.

By comparison, in Europe there is not the legal infrastructure to accommodate this type of company, nor are there people like him visible in the industry. Instead there are many hedonists partying hard or taking it easy in their sunset years. Those who don't smoke now, used to smoke before. Spannabis is Europe's largest cannabis trade show. In 2015, Spannabis held the World Cannabis Conferences in an adjoining building. They invited American speakers providing inside analysis on the cannabis economy, new regulations and business advice. The Hall was almost empty. Everyone was too busy partying and selling wares next door. Farrell was adjusting slowly to Europe's old-style approach. 'They are only into their Human Rights to consume—they don't actually offer anything' he told me.

This is not strictly true. There is much marketing of medical cannabis. Indeed, people that I've been speaking to are changing how they see cannabis. One woman said, 'I've always had a smoke before I go to bed, I thought it was fun but now I realise it helps me sleep'. Someone else said, 'When I used get stressed I wondered whether to smoke and forget about it or work out my feelings without weed. But [now] I can see that it is a medicine so tend to medicate myself'.

Nevertheless, the US business ethos has not carried through. The medicalisation of the discourse on cannabis has been adopted by the industry, albeit with occasional cynical marketing; for example, Caviar Gold promotes itself as the 'Strongest Medicine in the World'. One American cannabis entrepreneur was advising people, 'Never refer to marijuana—always say medical marijuana', but, by comparison with the US, Europe has been slow to catch on.

Large scale storage, medicalisation, and US health concerns about smoking, have helped drive the development of cannabis concentrates. By 2015, in addition to vaping fluids, popular additions to the cannabis trade included little dropper bottles, or needleless syringes, filled with tinctures and oils of THC, CBD or blends of selected cannabinoids. By 2016, marketing and products were extending to turpenes as well. One producer of medical oils told me that recent technology to blend different cannabinoids allowed for a vast array of different combinations of compound and dose, producing a multitude of potential products. Degrees of quality in cultivation and processing, he said, also affected user experience. Technological developments, like other innovations, provide greater sales possibilities and give competitive advantage. New products are sold into a differentiated market distinguished by cost, quality and quantity.

Research into cannabinoids is not restricted to the institutional laboratory governed by a history of disciplinary discussion and management committees. Research and development on cannabis, and the concentration of cannabinoids, is also a cottage industry; for some it is a proud artisan craft. The extraction of cannabinoids increases the purity and so supports the standardisation of treatments and medical trials. A product of about 99% pure THC is available. The medicalisation of cannabis is helping to develop concentrates of active compounds of cannabis. What we don't know yet is how that will change the culture of current cannabis using communities or groups. Although the modern history of coca does not provide a comparative model to predict social changes, like the shift from coca to cocaine, medicalisation and accompanying concentrates are changing the profile of the original plant substantially.

In the more institutionalised sectors of university research laboratories and global pharmaceuticals, cannabis is not the magic bullet evangelised by the needs of cannabis reformers, media hype and industry marketing. Instead it is another drug amongst many undergoing research, trial and development—mostly in conjunction with existing remedies. Allopathic medicine is less attached to the herbal origins of the plant than the chemistry derived from it. Research scientists I've spoken to are not set on using herbal cannabis to obtain cannabinoids. Chemically identical synthetic cannabinoids might offer a more cost effective and standardised alternative over herbal derivatives.

Products like GW Pharma's *Sativex*, while legally protected, are too easy to copy, especially with such a large cottage industry. Sativex already has strong competition from the illegal market in terms of similar products at lower costs and possibly better quality (though without the same rigours of standardisation, medical trials or legal protections). For big pharma to operate in cannabis markets they either need more effective prohibition, which is hard without popular consensus, or more sophisticated cannabis-based drugs.

Cannabis medicine is currently of far greater importance to the cannabis industry than the pharmaceutical industry. The Medical Cannabis Bike Tour is a novel funding stream in an area of marginal medical interest. What the cannabis industry and activists want is the development of cannabis medicine of herbal origins, preferably without piggy backing it onto existing chemotherapies. When medical institutions participate in this sort of development, they fortify the legitimacy of cannabis; the previously dangerous object can circulate more easily. In this scenario, cannabis contributes to society by healing unproductive bodies, saving healthcare costs, increasing economic output and all sanctioned by the current dominant scientific medical model.

Increasing legalisation also means greater potential collaborative partnerships between scientific R&D and the cannabis industry. Collaboration will depend on the quality of skills in a cannabis sector that has historically relied on marketing over integrity. Unlike other horticultural fields of expertise, cannabis seed breeders are the superstars of the cannabis world; they travel, promote product and their egos rage. One horticulturalist told me that cannabis genetics are not that well developed in comparison to other industries. Meanwhile, key strains and well-known brands are in the front line to be bought out by big money.

While the big money steps forward to claim the legal rights and infrastructures for tomorrow's markets, the plurality of legislations and local prohibition practices across Europe change with astonishing speed. What is legal one day may be illegal the next. A small family firm, and years of investment, can become illegal overnight as the line of the law moves. Seeds and growing equipment are in the forefront of changing governmental approaches. In Amsterdam one business owner said, 'They cannot wait to close us down. I now have to see a lawyer to find out if the employees are going to be liable if there is a problem'.

Entrepreneurs who see their competitors shut down by the state sit and wait for the same to happen to them. What they are allowed to sell has been greatly reduced but the government does not offer to compensate them for loss of business nor assist them in meeting new regulations. It is an exercise of power that has little consideration for how these people will meet their existing economic commitments. Inevitably, some of those who fail to adjust to the new legal regime will adjust to the new illegal one. The Dutch cannabis sector emerged as a consequence of legal measures to contain the dirt and danger associated with the circulation and consumption of the plant. As such it always shared a space with other economies similarly inscribed, that is, criminal productive activity. The move from legal regulated trading to illegal unregulated trading will, for some, be quite simple.

Most of the people I have spoken to in the industry, however, put enormous energy into trying to stay within the law. Some have migrated to Spain and the United States, others spend time and money re-marketing products to comply with the law. The view of danger and subversive behaviour is often misplaced. These businesses work very hard travelling the trade show circuits of Europe, United States and South America. They try to stay legal in a business made risky by unstable, fragmented regulation that sometimes widens sales opportunities and at other times closes them down.

As the US market grows and builds a strong infrastructure of production, transportation, investment and regulation, some of their European competitors are struggling to sustain its businesses. Connections with sanctioned wealth of government and pharmaceuticals contracts may not only be the route to riches, it could become the only means of legal survival.

The dominant politico-legal-medical-moral discourse often obscures the view of cannabis as produced, circulated and consumed in a variety of economic forms. The illegality of cannabis produces socially embedded trading through production–intermediary-consumer networks. Illegal cannabis is not an alienated product but is circulated through gift relations and fluid vendor-purchaser roles.[10] Similarly, alternative medicine has a far greater degree of forging personal relations in treatment than mainstream allopathic models. Medical cannabis within alternative medicine is more aligned to illegal cannabis circulations than pharmaceutical developments. It sits in the cross-over between non-personal cash exchange and building close social relationships as part of treatment. Yet, in the future, alternative medicine cannabis practitioners are more likely to end up in a space of legal transgression than the global pharmaceuticals because the hierarchy of legal transgression is, in part, build upon a hierarchy of societal institutions.

The cannabis economy gaining media attention is an aggressive capitalism based upon investment for monetary profit, product proliferation, and the creation of market opportunities. When we hear about the cannabis economy on the news they are not referring to the forms of gift exchange or exchanges based in establishing strong social ties. Instead, the cannabis boom assigned greater legitimacy by the media relates to the influx of stock market and venture capital. This moment of drug liberalisation follows a contemporary corporate model.

It will be in the interests of this growing industry to generate positive stories and positive web presence. They want to widen marketing targets and encourage us to consume more weed—cannabis will never have seemed so good. For a non-addictive drug, a lot of people already use it very regularly. People and cannabis develop remarkably dependent relationships together. Research shows how the gambling industry controls much of the knowledge production on gambling,[11] that is why we think there are individual problem gamblers rather than an industry devising ways of getting people to gamble more. I cannot think of a reason why a legitimate cannabis industry would behave any differently, after all any industry aims to sustain or increase consumption.

CONCLUSION

As cannabis becomes a more alienated commodity, dis-embedded from the social relations of illegal trading, we will find enjoyment in distinguishing our own consumer preferences in a differentiated market, just as we do when deciding between goods in Tesco's 'Everyday Value' and 'Finest' ranges. For a niche market, preferences will be influenced by marketing narratives designed to write off the gap between producer and consumer, for example, when buying a Fairtrade product from an organic farm in Patagonia.

As we embrace that market more, we live an increasingly commoditised life while drugging up to avoid the stress and alienation produced by the same commoditised style of living. We are aware of the problems of pharmaceutical industries but cheer on the new cannabis dispensaries as if they are benign and beneficial models of economy. Although some might worry about the implications on our bodies when taking medicines through big pharmaceuticals, a regular dose of cannabis does not enter into the framework because it currently occupies the same political space as opposition to the pharmaceutical industry. Cannabis is becoming the commoditised panacea of the counter-chemical movement. When the plant is taken from its original herbal form, genetically modified and specific chemical compounds extracted from it to make concentrates in an expanding multi-million dollar industry, we should step back for a moment. Why the rush to medicate with cannabis?

Cannabis has socio-political meaning that is not confined to prohibition debates. You might think that the world of psychedelics would take you away from a commoditised culture, let you see what was happening to this world and change it. Yet, when the consumption of cannabis is made more accessible, it becomes more work and entertainment within the same confines as before. Cannabis is part of the leisure and bodily repair sectors.

Cannabis is fragmenting into a variety of products while the international drug regulations are fragmenting into a variety of practices. The meanings that we ascribe to cannabis, and to our interactions with cannabis, will always take place within our culturing of particular forms of economy. The vast majority of people who create the cannabis industry (producers, regulators, seed breeders etc.) do not run alternative economic models or radically different ways of life, instead they chase the same golden goose. Cannabis becomes another commodity regulated by state and industry alliances. Nevertheless, short of substantial drug policy reform, there will always be areas of cannabis production and circulation that remain illegal. As mentioned earlier, Parry and Bloch considered an essential value for sustained reform was giving something back to society that reinforced central moral values. Unfortunately, in the context of drug reform, that becomes the sanctioned and complete assimilation into the political and economic values of the dominant form of political economy.

References:

1. Cross, S. 'Under a cloud: morality, ambivalence and uncertainty in news discourse of cannabis law reform in Great Britain'. In *Drugs and Popular Culture: Drugs, media and identity in contemporary culture*. Manning P, (ed). Routledge. 2013. 134–49.

2. Douglas, M. *Purity and Danger: An Analysis of Concepts of Pollution and Taboo*. London: Routledge. 2002.

3. Carpentier, C., Laniel, L., Griffiths, P. *Cannabis Production and Markets in Europe*. Lisbon: Office for Official Publications of the European Communities. 2012.

4. Roitman, J.L. *Fiscal Disobedience: An Anthropology of Economic Regulation in Central Africa*. Princeton University Press. 2005.

5. Arce A., Long, N. 'Consuming Modernity: mutational processes of change'. In *Anthropology, Development, and Modernities: exploring discourses, countertendencies, and violence*. Arce, A., Long, N., (eds). London: Psychology Press. 2000. 159–83.

6. Parry, J., Bloch, M. *Money and the Morality of Exchange*. Cambridge: CUP. 1989.

7. Hugh-Jones, S. 'Coca, Beer, Cigars and Yagé: Meals and Anti-Meals in an Amerindian Community'. In *Consuming Habits: drugs in history and anthropology*. Sherratt, A., Goodman, J., Lovejoy, P. (eds). London: Routledge. 1995. 47–66.

8. Princen, T. 'Consumption and its externalities: Where economy meets ecology'. In *Confronting Consumption*. Princen, T., Maniates, M., Conca, K. (eds). Cambridge: MIT Press. 2002. 23–42.

9. Blackman, S. *Chilling out: The cultural politics of substance consumption, youth and drug policy*. McGraw-Hill International. 2004.

10. Chatwin, C., Potter, G. 'Blurred Boundaries The Artificial Distinction Between 'Use' and 'Supply' in the UK Cannabis Market'. *Contemporary Drug Problems*. 2014 41(4):536–50.

11. Cassidy, R. 'Fair game? Producing and publishing gambling research'. *International Gambling Studies*. 2014 14(3):345–53.

THE GAIA PROJECT: RESTORING ANCIENT MYSTERIES

CARL A.P. RUCK

The ancient testimony about the religious experience offered to thousands of pilgrims in the sanctuary of the Goddess in the tiny village of Elefsina (Eleusis) some eleven miles west of the great city of Athens is unanimous. The Homeric Hymn to Demeter declares that it was essential to the art of living: 'Whoever among men who walk the earth has seen these Mysteries is blessed, but whoever is uninitiated and has not received his share of the rite, he will not have the same lot as the others, once he is dead and dwells in the moldering tomb beyond where the sun goes down.' The initiates were sworn to secrecy and the event was termed a Mystery. The rite was performed annually for two thousand years, beginning in the mid second millennium BCE, in roughly the same place, modified and enlarged over the course of time to accommodate the ever-growing number of participants. Construction of the sanctuary obliterated the archaeological record of the earlier occupation of the site, but it is probable that it was sacred from Neolithic times, if not before.

In the sixth century BCE, it passed under Athenian control and became the defining influence that produced the mentality that characterised the Classical Age, which became the fountainhead of ensuing European civilisation. Almost everyone of importance, as well as the common man and woman, foreigner and Greek alike of every status in society, sought out the initiation at least once in a lifetime. In the Roman period, the orator and philosopher Cicero declared it the greatest gift of Athens to the world, the essential impetus for humankind's elevation from savagery, imparting the power not only to live with joy, but also to die with better hope. 'For among the many excellent and indeed divine institutions which your Athens has brought forth and contributed to human life, none, in my opinion, is better than those Mysteries' (Cicero, *De legibus*, 2.14.36).

Eleusis was named like Elysium, a mirror of the paradisiacal fields (*Les champs Élysées*) that received the dead upon their arrival in the otherworld. It was sacred to the Goddess and her daughter, the two holy females, the 'Mother' and the 'Maiden,' who could be ascribed names, after the patriarchal revision that established the Classical version of the Mystery, as Demeter and Persephone, although more sacredly, they were just the two nameless goddesses (*tó theó*), interchangeable as mother produced daughter and daughter in turn became mother. The male essential for their replication was the personification of the joyous shout of the initiates as they walked in procession to the place of arrival, *Iácchos* – a punning calque upon the word for 'drug or toxin' (*ia-trós*, 'druggist') and upon the deity who led the ecstatic procession along the Sacred Road from Athens toward Elefsina, Dionysus/Bacchus, the god of wine and intoxicants, strongly suggesting that an altered consciousness was necessary to access the Mystery. He was identical here with his chthonic persona as Hades, the lord of the netherworld, named as the 'unseen one,' which was also the name for the invisible realm into which the living disappeared upon their arrival in the luxurious fields of the otherworld paradise.

A third female shadowed the personae of the two goddesses. The postmenopausal, but still nursing mother, who went by the dread name of Hecate, the patroness of witchcraft, who fed the living with the milk intended for her dead child. But all three roles were interchangeable, since the mother could become the wet nurse of the daughter's child, and it was this third that joined the two holy ladies into a triumphant trinity. In her iconography, she was represented by three young women, back to back, holding sacred emblems of the initiation.

The paradigm uniting life and death was the seed implanted into the ground, entrusted to the darkness of the earth, in the expectation that it would return and sprout, without which there could be no life here in the realm above. The initiates experienced a journey of the spirit to a reality in a parallel dimension, establishing pathways of communication and rights of friendly reciprocal visitation, so that life was nourished by the accord or testament that defined the terms for humankind's relationship to Gaia. It was more than a mere metaphor. The initiates were offered the opportunity to identify themselves with the most basic cycles of nature at the deepest level of their existence.

The mystery of the seed reborn was personified as the son born from the holy trinity, which had the mystery title of the Lady named *Brímo*, the terrible queen-ship. He was their child, named after them in matriarchal fashion as *Brímos*, but he had another less frightful name befitting the benevolence of this trinity as the 'triple warrior,' *Triptólemos*. It was he who was entrusted with the art of living and he planted the first crop in the surrounding Rarian fields. He was the pacified antithesis to the psychoactive toxic analogues of his parentage, life born from death. He was also named for the *trípolos*, the sacred field whose inaugural ploughing, repeated symbolically as an annual rite, required restitution in the form of some offering to Gaia to compensate for the intrusion of the phallic ploughshare into the furrow of Earth's vulva, by which the wilderness was converted to cultivation. The first ploughman was offered as sacrificial victim.[1] In the myth of the Mystery, he was represented by his brother *Demophóön* ('victim offered in the name of the people'), the child whose mortality Demeter had attempted to burn off in the fire of the hearth. In honour of him, each year a child from Athens was initiated at public expense.

The great hall of initiation at Eleusis was an architectural similitude of a cave, whose antiquity as a motif can be traced back to the Palaeolithic when humans first rose above the beasts as *Homo spiritualis*, not *sapiens*, but with the first inklings of spirituality, a remembrance of forgotten dreams.[2] The cave was the womb of Gaia, the vulva to a world beyond and a gateway for birth into this realm of ordinary living. Plato used the ancient motif as his Allegory of the Cave (Plato, *Republic*, 514a–520b). What the cavernous hall of the *Telesterion* offered was release from the Cave of ordinary seeing.

The initiates on the night of the great Mystery rematerialised in the hall of the sanctuary, after their spiritual journey to Elysium, at the moment of the miraculous birth of this primordial ploughman. They experienced themselves reborn, like him, a child conceived and born from death and destined like him to return to his chthonic family. The valence of death became positive through personal experience, and the lord Hades was recognised as a handsome youth of 'good counsel' (*Euboúleus*) and as the source of prosperity (personified as *Ploútos*) in both this real realm and the next.

What we know of the Mystery dates largely from the seventh century BCE, the probable date of the Homeric Hymn and its subsequent incorporation under Athenian control, but its origins go back at least to the mid-second millennium. Like all the great ancient religious sites of the Classical world, it represents an assimilation of a pre-existent sanctuary to the evolving dominance of the Indo-European Greek-speaking peoples, who migrated into the Mediterranean lands with their family of twelve Olympian deities, headed by the patriarchal father god Zeus.

In deference to this earlier existence of the religion, Demeter, who will teach the Mystery to *Triptólemos*, claims that she has come from Minoan Crete when she first arrives at Eleusis. Hades had abducted her daughter, begotten by her brother Zeus, while picking flowers with a sisterhood of maidens. The spiritual rapture experienced as an abduction is a common mythological motif, and involves always the special fantasies of herb cutters, the gatherers of magical plants or entheogens. Such plants are toxic and grow wild, and the maiden is abducted, not married to the possessing spirit that materialised from the magical plant.

A myth is read as a dialogue in the language established by its structural polarities. With the institution of the Mystery, Persephone has become the wedded wife of her abductor, transitioning from matriarchal independence among a sisterhood of females into sequestered seclusion within the household dominated by her husband. The abduction is associated with fleabane, the concubine of Hades. She was named *Mínthe* (*Mentha pulegium*), pennyroyal, which is an abortifacient and a toxic insecticide. As wife, Persephone has replaced her womb's aborted offspring with the parturition of her child. The abduction is also associated with the magical flower called *nárkissos* ('narcotic'), and narcosis, as induced by opium, is symbolic of death. The association of the opium poppy with the pre-Indo-European Minoan goddess is well documented, as well as the triple personae of her identity within a sisterhood of females. Furthermore, not only does abduction yield to marriage, but through death, Persephone yields life. She eats a seed of pomegranate as she leaves the underworld and becomes pregnant with Hades' son. The pomegranate resembles the opium poppy capsule, but signifies the fertile womb instead of death. Its name in Greek (*rhóa*) identifies the seedy red matrix of its fruit with the bloody 'flux' of the menses. Persephone with the pomegranate and scenes of her abduction were common motifs on sarcophagi.

Persephone should have been an Olympian, since both her mother Demeter and her father Zeus are Olympians, but she contaminated her eternal spiritual essence with physical matter since she has taken food and seed in the underworld, so that she now belongs like humans partially to her husband's world. Demeter becomes the mother-in-law of Hades and has a grandson as the Mystery child born from the chthonic realm.

I was a member of a team in the 1970s that sought to uncover what actually happened in the Eleusinian sanctuary.[3] It is well-documented that the experience was visionary, and that it had been profaned toward the end of the fifth century BCE by inducing it unlawfully among groups of revellers at private drinking parties by employing the sacred entheogen as a recreational drug. We demonstrated that the initiates were afforded a glimpse into a transcendent reality by the ingestion of a powerful psychoactive agent derived from ergot (*Claviceps purpurea*) a natural substance similar to LSD (lysergic acid diethylamide), LSA (lysergic acid amide), the same toxin that is the active agent in *ololiuqui*, as derived from certain morning glories in Mesoamerican shamanism, and apparently also known in ancient Greece and to European folkloric tradition as bindweed.

The initiates for the ceremony drank a special potion, called the kykeón or 'mixture,' whose ingredients in water as recorded in the Homeric Hymn were the wild fleabane and the cultivated barley. It was intended as a magical mediation of all the mythical structural polarities. It obviously should be something visionary or an entheogen, which neither the wild nor the cultivated ingredients are. Some, who admit that an intoxicant seems indicated, have assumed that the barley had fermented into a beer, but grain will not ferment unless it is mashed to convert its starch into fermentable sugar, and the indications of the episode of the profanations in Attic comedy make clear that the barley kernels were intact. A recent commentator suggests that the few raw barley kernels with an insecticide was intended as a nourishing meal to end the fast of the candidates for the initiation.[5]

A common weed in fields of grain provides the answer, tares or darnel, and perfectly fits the structural parameters established by the myth. Darnel is not grown as an edible grain crop, but it is an invasive wild grass in ploughed land, named as *Lolium temulentum*, the specific botanical Latin nomenclature designating it as 'drunken' because it always is infested with the fungal parasite of ergot, whose toxins were recognised as causing altered eyesight or hallucinations. Darnel's toxicity, however, derives solely from the ergot parasitic upon it. It is not toxic in itself. Grain from which the kernels of darnel were not sufficiently extracted was apparently made into a cheap kind of bread that caused one to see things that were not there. Its exclusion from the harvested crop was also ritualised in the Roman festival of the *Robigalia* by the offering of a sacrificial red dog, analogous to the primordial ploughman, symbolic of its wild persona, to free the fields of the invasive contamination. Ergot's red colour is responsible for its common name as 'rust,' *robiga* in Latin and *erysíbe* in Greek. With this metaphor, it is involved in the mythical account that the rust from the knife employed in the sacrificial offering of the primordial plough-land was a medicinal cure for the impotency of a king's son, who thought that his father was going to make him the human victim. In contrast to the abortifacient fleabane, ergot was employed by midwives to control postpartum bleeding. The goddess Demeter had the epithet of *Erysíbe*. The Latin equivalent was *Robigus*, who had a female analogue as *Robiga*. They presided over diseases of agriculture, capable of alleviating the rusting maladies they caused through the offering of the dog's red blood.

In the context of the mediation between the wilderness and the cultivated field and between lethal and edible foods, darnel (often called 'false wheat') was considered a wild weed that like a disease could attack the cereal grains and, as such, it was thought to have the potential to reverse the hybridisation of the edible crop back to the primordial or primitive grasses. The spread of the fungal infection from the darnel to the planted crop, and particularly to the barley, which seemed most susceptible to the infestation, was a clear demonstration of its recidivist threat. The most primitive of the cultivated grains from which barley was hybridised is spelt (*Triticum spelta*), mythologised as the food of olden days, which originally had only two red kernels or 'split' spikelets (hence its name). These resemble the protruding ergot spikes as they appear on barley, darnel, and the other grasses.[6] Like most grasses, spelt, too, is infested with ergot, and like darnel, spelt was seen as the primitive weedy antecedent of the hybridised superior cultivated grains, fruiting with only the two kernels, whereas the hybridised grasses like barley produce an entire sheaf or cob.

Ergot is easily recognisable as fungal inasmuch as the infested grain kernels host the mycelium or root-like growth that permeates and enlarges the kernel, and when it falls to the ground, it sprouts into the fruiting stage as little clearly discernible mushrooms, making the ergot-infested kernel seem to be the seed for the otherwise totally wild and uncultivatable mushroom. The mushroom's propagation by microscopic spores was unknown in antiquity, and hence the ergot, as a mushroom seed, seemed to mediate perfectly between the wild and cultivated plants.

The mushroom, furthermore, was seen as a 'fermentation' of the earth, and hence it partook of the whole symbolic complex of intoxicating fermented beverages and the leavening of bread. The two fundamental foods of humankind, the dry and the liquid, were paired as the gifts of Demeter and Dionysus. The wine of Dionysus was similarly involved in the ethnobotanical motif of wild and cultivated vines, with the grapevine and the civilised or sophisticated intoxicant yielded by fungal growth contrasted to the primitive vines, which resembled the grapevine, but are toxic in their natural state. These were the ivy and similar vines like bryony (wild cucumber) and smilax (wild morning glory, bindweed). The red colour of the ergot also associated it with particular red psychoactive mushrooms and the whole complex of ritual lycanthropy and the wolf's canine analogues, in particular the pelt of the red fox. The entire fox pelt was worn as the original version of the Phrygian cap, and the pointed snout of the fox was imitated in the felt hat. In European folkloric tradition, the ergot was caused by the grain mother passing like a wind rustling through the field with her pack of grain wolves (*Roggenwulf, Roggenhund*) infecting the sheaves of ergot or *Tolkorn* ('mad corn kernels'). Children seduced by goblin creatures into the fields nurse on the kernels like the iron teats of the *Roggenmutter* and are rendered maddened. The enlarged ergot infected kernels are called 'wolf teeth' (*Wulfzahn*). The Phrygian cap and its motif of lycanthropy occur in the folkloric tale of 'Little Red Cap', *Rotkäppshen*, known in its English version, which predates the collection of the Grimm brothers, as 'Little Red Riding Hood,' whose hood indicates that she is on a journey of symbolic significance.[7]

Thirty years after our initial unveiling of the Eleusinian Mystery, I returned to the subject to present a clearer explanation, incorporating many of these new discoveries made in the intervening years.[8] When I asked my colleague, the Swiss chemist Albert Hofmann, shortly before his death at the age of 102 to provide a comment, even if only a sentence, in view of his frailty, he wrote: 'Only a new Eleusis could help mankind to survive the threatening catastrophe in Nature and human society and bring a new period of happiness.'

Hofmann's discovery of LSD in 1943 was an event that inaugurated a new awareness of our role in the cosmos, and looking back at the end of the century whose mentality he, probably more than anyone, influenced, he saw the crisis that we humans have created by our destruction of our planet Gaia and the possible extinction of our species. By a new Eleusis, he was proposing to heal the dangerous separation of humankind's individual consciousness from its natural immersion in the surrounding environmental universe, which Nietzsche had characterised as the opposition between Apollonian and Dionysian modes of cognition.[9]

Elefsina is a place particularly blessed by Nature, a fertile plain bounded by mountain ranges surrounding the acropolis. The initiation hall was carved like a cave from the rock face of its southern slope, and marked as sacred by its alignment to the depression between the twin peaks called the 'Horns' (Kerata) that terminate the mountain to the west. Such alignment is typical of other Minoan and Pelasgian religious sites and identified the sanctuary by a sexual metaphor as the entrance, nestled between the breasts and spread legs of the bovine Goddess, to the secrets that lay within her body. It was here in the surrounding plain that barley, the grain plant that was the staff of life, first sprouted. The place was further blessed topographically by the island of Salamis that lies nearby along its shore, providing a superlative nearly land-locked shelter for ships in its bay. Most people know of it only from the account of the Battle of Salamis (480 BCE), when the Athenian admiral in charge of the allied fleet used his knowledge of the lay of the land to his advantage against the vastly superior forces of the invading Persian King Xerxes.

These blessings and the prosperity of the Eleusinian plain were also an invitation to abuse its natural gifts after the desecration of the sanctuary and the supplanting of its religion by the modern world. It is today a microcosm for the destruction that has spread around the planet—the catastrophe that looms threatening continued human existence. The bay of Salamis is clogged with tankers waiting to offload their cargo of crude oil to the mainland refineries that belch an air-polluting stench. The plain has dried into a desert that supports little agriculture. In addition to the refineries, two other industries process material wealth ravished from the earth, a cement factory and a foundry for iron. The cement factory until just recently has even been digging away at the backside of the Acropolis hill to convert its rock into useable cement and it owns the site of the bronze-age settlement on the summit, precluding its archaeological excavation. It is likely that many of the stones missing from the sanctuary suffered a similar fate. The symbolism could not be more obvious.

Few people now visit the sanctuary, or know of the ancient Mystery. Elefsina is not in the register of places recognised as a world heritage site, even though it was the center of a religion practiced for two millennia. The inadequate museum dates from the nineteenth century, and several of its treasures have been substituted with replicas. An effort is underway to improve the situation. The superhighway to Corinth now skirts the site, and the progressive local governments have worked to restore the village, with the streets around the sanctuary converted into pedestrian malls. The shore is planted with parklands and the sea is again clean enough for swimming. A large area of ruined and abandoned nineteenth-century factories adjacent to the sanctuary and below the present museum has been converted into a center for workshops and galleries for the display of art and theatrical performances.

As the place most desecrated for its abuse of Gaia, we propose that Elefsina become the nucleus and world center for humankind's renegotiation of its compact with its planet Earth. To this end, we are seeking recognition of the village and the archaeological remains as a world heritage site and are soliciting funding from international and Greek donors to build a new museum complex, incorporating the area and some of the abandoned industrial ruins that now comprise the art center. The symbolism is simple. We do not propose to restore a defunct religion or to reverse the course of time, but to begin anew with a new contract with Gaia. As in antiquity, we depend on the bounty of Gaia for prosperity.

The museum complex would be multifunctional. One of its tasks would be to investigate ways of mitigating the deleterious effects of exploiting natural resources. Industrial constructions are actually works of extraordinary complexity and ingenuity. At the new Elefsina, they will learn to operate cleanly, and surrounded by parklands they can be seen as monuments, gigantic sculptural testimony, functioning efficiently and beautiful, as their modern designers conceived them.

In addition to furthering research into the past and the study of the Eleusinian Mystery through seminars and conferences, the museum complex will look to the future. Among the sponsored activities will be investigations into rediscovering a personal commitment to Gaia through techniques of meditation, spiritual exercise, alternative medicine, and artist workshops. The center would also support research into environmental remediation and new sources of energy and safe methods of tapping the planet's gifts. Eventually we hope to see agriculture return to the Rarian plain, and make the museum a destination of pilgrimage again for the modern world.

The influence of the Thracian revisionist theology, attributed to Orpheus, added a new dimension to the Mystery tradition of Eleusis, which never really became officially incorporated into the Eleusinian tradition. After many returns, with purifying ordeals in both this world and the other, the incarnation would be nullified and the Apollonian spirit would ascend, divested of the burden of flesh, to its true home in the fiery empyrean beyond the stars for an eternal existence. That is the other alternative still today. The Earth polluted and desecrated of its bounty may require some few survivors to seek another home in the Cosmos.

References:

1. Ruck, C.A.P. *The Great Gods of Samothrace and the Cult of the Little People*. Berkeley, Regent Press. 2016.

2. Herzog, W. *Cave of Forgotten Dreams*. Documentary film of the Chauvet Cave discovered in 1994 in Southern France. Toronto Film Festival. 2010.

3. Wasson. R.G., Hofmann, A., Ruck, C.A.P. *The Road to Eleusis: Unveiling the Secret of the Mysteries*. New York: Harcourt Brace Jovanovich. 1978.

4. Webster, P., Perrine, D.M., Ruck, C.A.P. 'Mixing the Kykeon'. *Eleusis: J Psychoactive Plants Comp.* 2000 4:55–86.

5. Cosmopoulos, M. Bronze Age *Eleusis and the Origins of the Eleusinian Mystery.* Cambridge: Cambridge University Press. 2015.

6. Watkins, C. 'An Indo-European agricultural term: Lain ador, Hittite hat-.' Harvard stud class 1973 77:187–194.

7. Ruck, C.A.P., Staples, B.D., González Celdrán, J.A., Hoffman, M.A. *The Hidden World: survival of pagan shamanic themes in European fairytales.* Durham: Carolina Academic Press. 2007.

8. Ruck, C.A.P. *Sacred Mushrooms of the Goddess: Secrets of Eleusis.* Berkeley: Ronin Publishing. 2006.

9. Hofmann. A. 'The message of the Eleusinian Mysteries for today's world'. Wasson et al. *The Road to Eleusis: unveiling the secret of the Mysteries.* Los Angeles: Hermes Press. 1998. 141–149.

LUNAR MEANDERS: KNOWLEDGE AND POWER IN PSYCHEDELIC LANDSCAPING

DALE PENDELL

> ... *by characterizing it as other than himself,* [the presence was] *preserved, nourished, and secretly made strong.*
> —Salman Rushdie, *The Satanic Verses*

like gods, (the many) gods, budded off from the One, but then sovereign. (& the One, named, is already dyadic, born in fission.)

A certain subtle strength is required to keep all those angels at bay, that they come when called, and take siesta when not needed, yes,

because without that particular strength, which is really a kind of gentleness, they will move in and take over—

that is why it is a poison path.

So with all writing, and all creation.

∞∞∞∞∞∞∞

'If you say it, it won't happen.'

& other sayings regarding psychic landscapes
& the mysterious 'it'
    that transforms them.

Blake is worth quoting:
    The Eternal Body of Man is The Imagination
        God himself
    that is
        The Divine Body
    It manifests itself in his Works of Art (In Eternity All is Vision)
    —William Blake, *The Laocoön.*

Imagination
        clothes the trees,
        every thought palpable.

Trungpa called it 'super-samsara,'
& by its excess
        made plain.

∞∞∞∞∞∞

Psychedelic *thinking* is the integration of the insights gained from psychedelic experience with our everyday life.
    —Cameron Adams, in *Breaking Convention: Essays on Psychedelic Consciousness*

Philosophy declined
    at least for a while.
'Stock Market Report, Daily Californian, 1965:
    LSD   +3
    Existentialism   -2'

Many tried to grasp something fuzzy—
   "round yon virgin'?

or entered
   the dialectics of emptiness,
or sought vision
   and found a cleansing
and nurtured such
   to the core of a life.

The super-structure, of course,
misses by a mile—
   silhouettes, or shadow prints.
Like now...

∞∞∞∞∞∞

It's cold out there on snow-capped vision peak.

Many learned domestics.
Improved?
Perhaps.

It's cold out there on snow-capped vision peak.
But not on tropical fern-topped peak,
or in a temperate canyon
   filled with redwood shadow
all 'Self' reduced to
a green glowing, like a radioactive powder,
   self-luminescent,
and abiding there
   without definition:
Samadhi.
Or playing basketball.

∞∞∞∞∞∞

Psychedelic thinking is how we rationalise psychedelic insight/ experience. And, learned usually sooner than later, pithy adages are never quite on the mark. Seemingly inevitably. By their nature. As in 'The Tao that can be named is not the true Tao.' Some version of that.

It is consciousness itself, not what consciousness apprehends. Or, is it the apprehending? Or, is there consciousness apart from the act of apprehending?

But that turns out not quite to be *it* either. (Try this yourself.)

We keep forgetting.
Oh right, I forgot.
That grabbing anything (thought, object, insight) out of the stream, freezes it: Huxley's ice cubes.
    And that 'it' is not *the* it.

Or are we verging on monotheism?

Unless one is philosophically inclined, all of that can be ignored with advantage.

('I spent my whole trip dancing in front of a mirror.')

∞∞∞∞∞∞

It's hard to bring it back in words because, as in a dream, stuff keeps happening—and hanging onto the words alters the ongoing events— that is, being fully present, which is kind of close to *it*. Tricky, but not impossible. What I've been calling 'dimensional smuggling'—getting words back across the frontier.

∞∞∞∞∞∞

Focus
or
Distraction.
LSD is good at both.

∞∞∞∞∞∞

Even if we can't quite say what *it* is, with experience, we can learn to point to it. Is it that I am in tune with these birds, my mind-colours turning when they do? Or are the birds responding to my mind?

HOW DO THEY KNOW?!

Or both: birds and each of us here at the lake inseparably part of a greater awareness, the whole forest waking up together—singing, yelling, chirping, flying and flitting, as pink and orange light cracks the sky with tiny flashes like magnesium flares.

We know they know because we squeal and the birds squeal back.

But why is this dawning different? How do they know we're high? Is it our timing? As if we were following the same invisible conductor as the birds, and with enough precision that the birds give us a pass?

Or could we do this any morning,
as long as the neighbours didn't call the cops?

Bipeds on drugs—squealing and shouting like gibbons do when the sun comes out after a three-day storm.

∞∞∞∞∞∞

Ann and Sasha Shulgin slowed down the second hand on their clock, and then stopped it. And it's kind of like, 'you had to have been there.'

∞∞∞∞∞∞

Or like a poem, how we get them. 'Recollected in tranquility?' Yeah, done that too. But that's different from 'given.' As in gift, poison to the root: 'bride-price.' I give you my self/body/mind. My time. My life. To have, to breathe through, to inspire.

∞∞∞∞∞∞

One part of it is: the other stuff out there—the other beings: resonances, sovereignties, continuums, that may, or may not, pause to twinkle an eye or lift a hat.

I believe, this morning anyway, that the stuff is always out there, but that we are mostly too preoccupied to greet, or witness, or even to notice.

For scientific experiments, viable controls present a challenge. It has not, to my knowledge, been proved that such experiments are impossible, but the need for some subtlety is obvious enough.

Induction is best.

And comparison, and recollection, over a span of years, from a traditional and structured discipline, such as Zen Buddhism, can be helpful.

'It's like I'm walking over ground I saw from the air,' one said.

∞∞∞∞∞∞

Certain psychedelic insights may be the same as, or indistinguishable from, certain insights of mysticism. But context matters—if the insight is separated from its context it is not quite the same insight. It may, in fact, miss the point entirely. But a Zen insight, out of its context, may be as warped as a psychedelic insight out of context, or more so. You can't call one 'true' and the other 'false'. It's more about a way, a path, a method.

It may be true, however, that deep satori-like insights from LSD tend to be associated with 'specialness,' all that sparkle, a special state— 'expanded consciousness'—and are thus less likely to be integrated, to be taken seriously, in everyday life. Than say, an idea one got just sitting on a cushion.

But we keep forgetting.
In both cases.

Right now I can't even remember what it was I forgot.
Two young, recently fledged red-shouldered hawks are making fools of themselves, screeching like goshawks, or drunken seagulls. Sun spin. Me too.

PSYCHEDELICS, TRANSGRESSION AND THE END OF HISTORY

ALAN PIPER

> *(LSD) came to symbolize, in particular, the irreducible ambivalence,*
> *between negation and affirmation, destruction and construction, of*
> *any transgressive act or experience.*
> —H. Isernhagen, 'Acid Against Established Realities', (1993)

> *History is going to end. This is the astonishing conclusion I draw from*
> *the psychedelic experience.*
> —Terence McKenna, 'The Archaic Revival', (1991)

LSD and other psychedelics now stand in a curious position. Once revelling in their transgressive status, they now wish to 'to come in from the cold' and return from a period of isolation, concealment and exile to circles of deserved esteem. Ironically, drugs that were once the touchstone of alterity, when being hip meant 'had you turned on?', now seek the legitimacy of medical and scientific authority and legally recognised sacramental status. In my presentation on 'Psychedelics, Transgression and the End of History' I asked, against a background of enthusiasm for a current 'Psychedelic Renaissance', whether the commodification of psychedelics in the form of approved psychedelic medicines, necessarily provided by Big Pharma, and the licencing of psychedelics for spiritual purposes in formally recognised churches, meant psychedelics would 'lose their mojo'. That is to say, would they have lost the radically enlightening quality ascribed to them by the likes of Terence McKenna, whereby psychedelics supposedly deprogram the user from the meta-narratives of Church, State and consumer society that condition us to accept the status quo?

Since I spoke in July 2015, I have found two more useful sources exploring the same territory of psychedelics, transgression and oppositional culture. First, Isernhagen's 'Acid against Established Realities' (1993) and secondly Leung's 'Ecstasy and Transcendence in the Postmodern State' (2011). Isernhagen in particular supports the view that I propounded, namely that psychedelics were co-opted by a pre-existing culture of resistance to Modernity. According to Isernhagen:

> One might begin by asking why drugs acquired such cultural significance in the 1960s and 1970s at all. In my view this was because there already existed a well-established cultural tradition—that of aesthetic Modernism (ca. 1900/1910–?) which was searching for what one might term alternate realities: there also existed a well-established language to express this search and its results.

Both Isernhagen and Leung focus on the transgressive nature of psychedelics. Leung argues for the legitimisation of the religious aspects of psychedelic experience, and does this partly by reference to the transgressive nature of psychedelic experience. She argues that psychedelic experience promotes transcendent perspectives and values which transgress the dominant ideology of consumer capitalism, which places the highest value on rationality, logic, efficiency and productivity. Leung references, as I did, Taussig's essay on transgression (2006), which argues that transgression is precisely the place in which the sacred is to be found in modernity. Transgression as a path to the sacred has a long history, and when the conformity of orthodoxy fails to deliver we turn to the heterodox and heretical to renew our experience of the sacred. It is ironic that the Enlightenment deconstruction of the Christian faith, for example by revealing broad structural parallels of world-wide myths of origin and redemption, actually led to a resurgence of interest in the old gods of Greece, Egypt and Europe, the occult and Gnostic cults in a search for the numinous.

PSYCHEDELICS, TRANSGRESSION AND THE COUNTERCULTURE

Most accounts of the history of psychedelics and psychedelic culture look no further back than the 1960s in terms of origins. Accounts also tend to be framed around the impact of appearance of psychedelics on society, whether in the visual arts, music or literature as well as spurring oppositional political movements. My intention here, against the common approach, is to look at the way in which psychedelics were embraced, understood and employed as a 'technology of resistance' by a pre-existing oppositional movement in 20th century culture. That is to say, how existing subcultural streams affected the way in which psychedelics were adopted, understood and employed in a positive sense, rather than their usual framing as the object of resistance by a status quo which demonised them and their celebrants.

As early as 1948, when LSD was hardly known even in the scientific community, the prominent German author and drug adventurer Ernst Jünger wrote to Albert Hofmann about Hofmann's reports to him concerning LSD: 'It seems indeed that you have entered a field that contains so many tempting mysteries... These are experiments in which one sooner or later embarks on truly dangerous paths, and may be considered lucky to escape with only a black eye'. Later, in 1961, but still well before psychedelics had achieved the kind of popularity among the youth of developed counties that made them the subject of a moral panic, Albert Hofmann expressed to Ernst Jünger his concern over the possible transgressive nature of psychedelics in these terms:

I must admit that the fundamental question very much occupies me, whether the use of these types of drugs, namely of substances that so deeply affect our minds, could not indeed represent a forbidden transgression of limits.

According to drug historian Marcus Boon (2006):

The words 'drugs' and 'literature" in their modern senses both emerged around the same time (circa 1800, with the Romantics)... And both become... places filled with an allure that is all the more intense because of the sense of the forbidden, of transgression, with which they are invested.

I think that these various remarks are sufficient to establish that psychedelics have what might be called an inherent aura of transgression; an aura that is dependant neither purely on their current illegality due to their supposed harmful effects, nor their supposed ability to foment a revolutionary discontent.

WHAT IS TRANSGRESSION?

What though is transgression or transgressive behaviour? By dictionary definition, transgression is defined as the violation of a law or a duty or moral principle or the action of going beyond or overstepping some boundary or limit. The concern expressed by Hofmann in 1961, given the then legal status of LSD, must have lain essentially in the second category. A transgressive action can be one of neglect or omission, but in terms of oppositional culture it often assumes the deliberate intention to shock, offend or harm another, but also includes:

- Acts that expose oneself to shocking or dangerous experiences with the possibility of mental or physical harm
- Acts of excess or greed, but also excessive and harmful abstinence

Acts of transgression tend to be those that damage or violate the integrity of a structure:

- The Mind
  Anything disruptive of normal mental processes or the sense of self
- The Body
  Cutting, mutilation, tattooing, scarification
- Society
  Socially disruptive acts, breaking local laws, customs or taboos
- The State
  Coup d'état, revolution, breaking national laws
- The Natural Order of Being
  The abnormal, the artificial or deviant
- The Sacred Order of Being
  The blasphemous, sacrilegious, taboo or impure
- A material thing for example a work of art or religious artefact
  Defacement, defilement or profanation

Such acts of transgression would include works of art that are disruptive and threaten to overturn the existing standards by which art is measured. Also, works of art that depict or describe an act of transgression or are themselves deliberately damaged, such as a deliberately corrupted text as in Burroughs' 'cut up' technique. Such acts can be playful, such as painting a moustache on the Mona Lisa or involve varying degrees of violence, such as performance art that involves self-mutilation.

TRANSGRESSION AS THE ESSENCE OF MODERNISM

Long before the psychedelic 60s, there was an oppositional culture that rejected the same aspects of 20th century Western culture that the countercultural revolutionaries of the 1960s later opposed. That opposition was to what are considered the characteristics of Modernity in Western industrialised states:

- Enlightenment Rationalism
- Capitalism/Consumer Culture/Commodification
- Industrialisation/Mass Production
- Institutionalised Religion
- Materialism
- The Enmity of Nation States

That oppositional culture promoted by way of opposition:

- The Irrational
  Dada/Surrealism
- Natural Living
  Rational dress/Ruralism/Vegetarianism
- Arts and Crafts
  William Morris/Ruskin
- Heterodox Gnosis
  Greek Mysteries/Christian Gnostic Cults
- Unseen Forces
  Spiritualism/Society for Psychical Research
- The Primitive and Exotic in Art
  Gauguin/Picasso
- Utopian Communities
  Oneida C19/The Farm C20

Largely expressed through the media of art, literature, music and film, this counter-movement has come to be termed 'Modernism' and its exponents 'Modernists', who somewhat confusingly were opposed to what is termed 'Modernity'. Those who opposed Modernity considered themselves to be heretics and Peter Gay's study of Modernism is subtitled 'The Lure of Heresy—From Baudelaire to Beckett and Beyond' (Gay, 2009). In 1909 a group of cutting-edge intellectuals in Cambridge formed what they termed The Heretics Society, whose lecture series included presentations by George Bernard Shaw (Literature), Ludwig Wittgenstein (Philosophy), Jane Harrison (Classics) and J.B.S. Haldane (Science).

TRANSGRESSION AS THE MODERN ENTRY POINT TO THE SACRED

For the Modernists, heresy and transgression were the points where individuals could find personal gnosis *versus* religious conformity and received wisdom, and an authentic existence *versus* social conformity. Illumination in this 'Counter Enlightenment' was sometimes sought by a deliberate derangement or bypassing of rational processes, though it had an ambiguous relationship with science and technology. Thus the famous quote by Rimbaud:

> The poet makes himself a seer by a long, prodigious, and *rational* disordering of all the senses... For he arrives at the unknown... and even if, crazed, he ends up by losing the understanding of his visions at least he has seen them!

At the same time, late 19th and early 20th century scientific developments emphasised the importance of unseen forces and an immaterial realm by reference to:

- Electricity
- X-Rays
- Quantum Physics
- Atomic Theory
- Darwinian Evolution
- Marxism
- Psychoanalysis

All of which depict surface appearances as the product of unseen forces, which can only be uncovered by and understood by initiates and explained using specialised technical language. Science was engaged in service of the search for proof of unseen forces, such as those providing for psychokinesis and telepathy, by the Society for Psychical Research, recalling Aleister Crowley's famous remark 'Our method is science, our aim is religion'.

Isernhagen notes 'the coincidental emergence of the modernist concern with alternate realities and the scientific exploration of those outskirts of the mind where religious and drug-induced experiences take place' in connection with the late 19th century investigations of William James into the mentally expanding effects of psychoactive drugs. The boundaries between personal and medical experimentation had yet to be clearly defined. Isernhagen notes the psychedelic 60s' 'dominant mode and mood were the same transgression of boundaries that characterizes the twentieth century's other avant-gardist innovations.'

Psychedelics were thus the ideal drug of Modernist aesthetic, intellectual and spiritual experimentation. They were disruptive of normal perceptions and forms of understanding, but provided for:

- Novel forms of perception and insight
- Deep self-examination
- An awareness of inner, normally unconscious processes
- An outward awareness of external universal processes

This explains their enthusiastic adoption as a key technology for transgressing normal limits of perception and experience by a pre-existing 'oppositional culture', and the suspicion and resistance of a status quo that placed a high value on rational, productive processes.

Chris Jenks in his examination of the culture of transgression argues that transgression 'has become the modern, post-God initiative, a searching for limits to break, an eroticism that goes beyond the limits of sexuality. God becomes the overcoming of God' (Jenks, 2003). In a similar vein, according to Michael Taussig (1996) 'Intoxication as an explosively dislocating and reconfiguring mystical force... is a dangerous territory, but one we cannot avoid in discussing transgression and modernity at the end of the twentieth century, with drugs as much if not more than sex occupying a strategic position in politics, revolution, counterrevolution and the sacred'. These statements reflect the belief of the Modernist movement that truth was to be found in the extremes of human experience, including the deliberate derangement of the senses, processes of free association and the outcome of random processes. Thus the exploration of dissonance in music that abandoned traditional notions of harmony, such as that of Béla Bartók (1881–1945), free jazz, and modern 'industrial genres'; the development of techniques of collage in art; the free associative and stream of consciousness text of James Joyce's *Ulysses* (1922) and the cut-up technique utilised by William Burroughs. The term 'stream of consciousness' was coined by Williams James in his *The Principles of Psychology* (1890), and later applied to a novel style in writing that reflected the naturalistic, free associative, stream of thought in a literary context, epitomised by James Joyce's Modernist novels. Thus the use of psychedelic drugs found a natural home in the environment of the Modernist aesthetics of the avant-garde and the positive interpretation of experiences under the influence of psychedelics, which could be and were also interpreted as typical of a disordered mind. In this way psychedelics became a 'technology of resistance' in service of the pre-existing 'oppositional consciousness' of Modernism and within countercultural circles of the 60s a touchstone of alterity. Hip versus Straight meant 'had you turned on?'.

ARE PSYCHEDELICS FUNDAMENTALLY TRANSGRESSIVE?

According to Terence McKenna; 'Psychedelics are illegal not because a loving government is concerned that you may jump out of a third story window. Psychedelics are illegal because they dissolve opinion structures and culturally laid down models of behaviour and information processing. They open you up to the possibility that everything you know is wrong.' This is an attractive idea and one that chimes with the notion that psychedelics fuelled the revolutionary 1960s. There must be truth in what McKenna claimed, because in the 1960s psychedelics without doubt became a tool of resistance to the status quo and icon of the counterculture. However, while the psychedelic experience may disabuse you of the metanarratives of Church and State there is no reason to assume that the new values adopted will be liberal. While they may be well tend to be 'libertarian', such values can swing to left or right.

Timothy Leary's theatrical celebration and promotion of psychedelics has been blamed for the illegal status of psychedelics and the end of medical research. If psychedelics had remained an interest only of intellectual elites, their status may well be different today. However, as agents with profound and sometimes confusing and disorientating psychological effects it appears unlikely that they would have indefinitely escaped becoming controlled substances. Even enthusiasts do not consider psychedelic experiences to be without any danger, and harm reduction is regularly on the agenda at Breaking Convention conferences. Timothy Leary (1963) wrote: 'Licensing will be necessary. You must be trained to operate. You must demonstrate your proficiency to handle consciousness-expanding drugs without danger to yourself or the public.'

Does McKenna's claim then overlook what nominally makes psychedelics fundamentally transgressive in social terms? Unfortunately governments' inability to distinguish between the different character of psychedelics and drugs such as heroin, amphetamines and cocaine impacts on their legal status. However, psychedelics do violate fundamental social values because:

- Derangement of the senses may be a danger to self
- Derangement of the senses may be a danger to others
- Irresponsible supplying of drugs may be a danger to others

It should be further observed that historically and transculturally the use of mind-altering drugs has usually been taboo and subject to ritual and restrictions, such as in the secrecy on pain of death regarding the Kykeon of Eleusis, and the dietary and other restrictions in use of Ayahuasca and Peyote. Strict rules usually determine who can and cannot use these powerful substances and when, where and for what reason and purpose.

'PSYCHEDELIC ESCHATON—BANG OR WHIMPER?' AND 'AFTER TRANSGRESSION WHAT?'

In his 'The Archaic Revival' Terence McKenna wrote 'History is going to end. This is the astonishing conclusion I draw from the psychedelic experience' (McKenna 1991). McKenna thus promoted an apocalyptic aspect to psychedelic culture, which borrowed significantly from the idea of an 'Omega Point' from the Jesuit priest Teilhard de Chardin (1881–1955) and initially focussed on the year 2012. McKenna envisaged his 'end of history' as a 'transcendental departure from business as usual' with psychedelics being the agency of immanentising a psychedelic re-visioning of society. The sense that Western culture was on a trajectory which would lead to its collapse was famously propounded by Oswald Spengler in his 'Decline of the West' (1918), where he wrote 'It would appear, then, that Western consciousness feels itself urged to predicate a sort of finality inherent in its own appearance'. I take McKenna's 'end of history', as with Spengler, to refer to our current cultural epoch and the initiation of a new cultural order. However, an 'end to history' could mean either the initiation of a new cultural epoch or that human society has reached its final state of cultural development and consciousness. An alternative conception of an 'end of history' has been proposed by Professor Fukuyama (2012), which he envisages as the global triumph of capitalism, liberal humanism, democracy and an end of competing ideologies; an infinite and peaceful extension of Western culture. While awaiting the arrival of McKenna's apocalyptic transition to a new order, what place for psychedelics in the increasing dominance of Fukuyama's consumer capitalism?

According to a review of Chris Jenks's study of the 20th century fascination with the power of transgression: 'Now that the twentieth century infatuation with transgression as an end in itself has lost much of its power, it is time to explore the sources and weigh the consequences of its disturbing appeal.' In the arts and modern media, acts of transgression occupied such a major role in the Modernist opposition to Enlightenment rationalism that transgressive acts in the arts became normalised, and cheap paperback copies of de Sade, Lautréamont and *The Story of O* appeared in the 1960s. Transgression has now moved from niche into the mainstream with the normalisation of hard pornography through the agency of the Internet and what has come to be termed 'torture porn' in the shape of films such as *Hostel*. Mark Dery asks, in his essay 'Been There, Pierced That' (2012), if we have become un-shockable and transgression has been commoditised and sold back to us not only as art, but as entertainment. Is transgression now 'so last century' and with that its socially and personally transformative power? In Peter Gay's study of Modernism (2008) he notes how avant-garde masterworks were 'absorbed into the very canon their authors professed to despise and had worked to discredit. With time, offensive (or at least startling innovations)... lost their power to outrage' and 'the absorptive capacity of a cultural establishment that modernists had worked so hard to subvert was nothing less than impressive'. Peter Gay is not the only author to have observed the capacity of capitalist culture to absorb, commoditise, sell back and thus neutralise the power of transformative agents. bell hooks, writing about the way in which interactions between racial identities and capitalism can perpetuate systems of oppression, makes a universally important point when she writes concerning the transformative power of something as simple as the symbolic power of styles of dress as agencies of resistance. 'As (agencies), their power to ignite critical consciousness is diffused when they are commodified' and 'Communities of resistance are (then) replaced by communities of consumption'. In that context I asked in 2015 what psychedelic communities of consumption might look like and suggested:

- The 'orthodox heresy' of Psychedelic Churches
- The medicalisation as NICE approved psychedelics provided by Big Pharma
- Drug tourism may in due course appear as a Thomas Cook 'Ayahuasca Journey'
- The merchandising of psychedelic culture as books, DVDs and T-Shirts
- Psychedelic conferences

In this scenario I asked the question: 'Have psychedelics lost their subversive mojo and been absorbed into an existing New Age "Spiritual Supermarket" and into a developing religious and medical orthodoxy?' In this connection I proposed three main domains of contemporary psychedelic culture.

- Medical & Scientific use and investigations of psychedelics
  In which psychedelics acquire medical and scientific meaning, but operate only within legal and professional restrictions
- Sacramental Psychedelia
  In which psychedelics are accepted as having religious meaning, but operate only within legal and doctrinal restrictions
- Pure or Recreational Psychedelia
  Which belongs to the sphere of personal consumption often expressed through music, art and literature in defiance of legal or other restrictions

I suggested that only in the realm of recreational psychedelia do psychedelics retain the power to subvert, challenge and transform.

Zieger in her prehistory of contemporary psychedelic culture (2008) considers the possibility that if 'like the mediations of the cinema and later, television, hallucinogens were amenable to the rhythms of bourgeois industrial life... they could be admitted into the legitimate sphere of bourgeois recreation' and then 'they could "transfigure" the world while leaving mind, body, and the status quo of workday life intact'. But she considers this to be the 'impossible promise' of the hallucinogens. Zieger concludes that the reason why, so far, hallucinogens have failed to become more popular and integrated into the rhythms of bourgeois life is, above all, because 'their seeming promise of intellectual transcendence meant that their dissemination through white, middle-class societies would threaten an imperial order keyed to racial, class, and gendered hierarchies'. And that they therefore 'remain more powerful as a fantasy of hidden knowledge'. I would argue that, once commodified as medicines or sacraments and subject to tight regulation, psychedelics are entirely amenable to the rhythms of bourgeois industrial life. However the unregulated and chaotic disordering of the senses, in search of otherwise hidden orders of being, will remain the domain of the artist and bohemian outsider.

There is no doubt that psychedelics fulfil a fundamental human desire and that desire can only be a desire for the dramatic but temporary overturning of our usual modes of understanding and perception, because that is the nature of psychedelic experience. According to Joan Cocks (1989):

> desire expresses itself most fully where only those absorbed in its delights and torments are present... it triumphs most completely over other human preoccupations in places sheltered from view. Thus it is paradoxically in hiding that the secrets of desire come to light, that hegemonic impositions and their reversals, evasions, and subversions are at their most honest and active, and that the identities and disjunctures between felt passion and established culture place themselves on most vivid display.

There is a deep human resistance to control in the desire to celebrate one's native being without external judgement or interference, a desire that is most powerfully catalysed by psychedelics outside of hegemonic cultural constraints.

Sources:

Boon, M. Foreword to Benjamin, W. *On Hashish*. Cambridge, MA: Harvard University Press. 2006.

Cocks, J. *The Oppositional Imagination*. London: Routledge. 1989.

Dery, M. 'Been There, Pierced That: Apocalypse Culture and the Escalation of Subcultural Hostilities'. In *I Must Not Think Bad Thoughts*. Minneapolis, MIN: University of Minnesota Press. 2012.

Fukuyama, F. *The End of History and the Last Man*. London: Penguin. 2012.

Gay, P. *Modernism: The Lure of Heresy*. New York, NY: W.W. Norton. 2008.

hooks, b. 'Eating the Other: Desire and Resistance'. In *Black Looks: Race and Representation*. Boston, MA : South End Press. 1992.

Isernhagen, H. 'Acid Against Established Realities: A Transcultural and Transdisciplinary View of LSD and Related Hallucinogens'. In *50 Years of LSD, Current Status and Perspectives of Hallucinogens*. Pletscher and Ladewig (eds). New York, NY: Parthenon Publishing Group. 1993.

Jenks, C. *Transgression*. London: Routledge. 2003.

Leary, T., Alpert, R. 'The Politics of Consciousness Expansion'. *Harvard Review*. 1963 1(4):33–37.

Leung, M. 'Ecstasy and Transcendence in the Postmodern State: The Search for Intimacy through Psychedelic Drugs'. 2011. Available at: https://amanitapieces.wordpress. com/2011/07/29/ecstasyand-transcendence-in-the-postmodern-state-the-search-for-intimacy-through-psychedelicdrugs/

McKenna, T. *The Archaic Revival*. San Francisco, CA: HarperSanFrancisco. 1991.

Spengler, O. *The Decline of the West*. New York, NY: Oxford University Press. 1991.

Taussig, M. 'Transgression'. In *Walter Benjamin's Grave*. Chicago, IL: University of Chicago Press. 2006.

Zieger, S. 'Victorian Hallucinogens'. Romanticism and Victorianism on the Net. No. 49, February 2008. Available at: http://id.erudit.org/iderudit/017857ar

THE PINEAL ENIGMA: LIFE AND TIMES OF THE 'DMT GLAND'

GRAHAM ST JOHN

Even Dr Gonzo would not touch 'extract of pineal'. It was the limit. 'One *whiff* of that shit would turn you into something out of a goddamn medical encyclopedia! Man, your head would swell up like a watermelon, you'd probably gain about a hundred pounds in two hours... claws, bleeding warts, then you'd notice about six huge hairy tits swelling up on your back...' He shook his head emphatically, 'Man, I'll try just about anything; but I'd never in hell touch a pineal gland.'[1] While Raoul Duke's Samoan attorney in *Fear and Loathing in Las Vegas* respectfully avoided the pineal, others have made this enigmatic gland, and its status as a possible brain site for the production of DMT (*N,N*-dimethyltryptamine), a *cause célèbre*. Remote from the misshapen grotesqueries conjured by Hunter S. Thompson, for clinical psychiatrist Rick Strassman the 'blinding light of pineal DMT' enables transit of the life-force from this life to the next. Such was the contention as published in Strassman's now popular book *DMT: The Spirit Molecule*, based on federally approved research at the University of New Mexico Hospital Clinical Research Centre, Albuquerque, between 1990–1995, in which he administered over four hundred IV doses of DMT to sixty healthy volunteers.

A relatively obscure compound at the time of *DMT: The Spirit Molecule*'s publication, Strassman's landmark study raised the profile of DMT, a potent short-lasting tryptamine known to effect out-of-body states, and to produce profound changes in sensory perception, mood and thought. While DMT is an integral component of the brew ayahuasca, it has an independent history and ontology, today inspiring an underground community of enthusiasts who typically embrace the 'entheogenic' (inner divinity awakening) propensities of this and other compounds. Likened to a gnosis event, and sometimes compared with a near-death experience, the DMT 'breakthrough' potentiates significant outcomes associated with perceived contact with 'entities' and the transmission of information often in the form of visual language.[2] With Strassman's book becoming a best seller, and with film-maker Mitch Schultz working with Strassman to produce a documentary film, also titled *DMT: The Spirit Molecule*—the Facebook page for which has nearly one million likes at the time of writing—Strassman's project has played a key role in this development.

But this is somewhat downstream from Strassman's project, at which time the noise on DMT had been restricted, tempered, and limited. Since 1956, when its psychopharmacology had been discovered by Stephen Szára, and psychiatrists had taken an interest in its psychotomimetic (psychosis mimicking) function, the science on DMT was limited to its possible role in psychoses. The situation was compounded by the War on Drugs, underway since the mid-1960s and thwarting research into the human experience with DMT (as it did with other psychedelics). Strassman's groundbreaking observations of the subjective effects of DMT on his volunteers constituted the first sanctioned research on the clinical application of psychedelics in the United States for a generation. Shining speculation on the phenomenal implications of DMT's endogenicity in human consciousness, *DMT: The Spirit Molecule* sparked a renewed wave of interest in the pineal gland, in which speculation and truth claims have often been conflated with truths.

THE SPIRIT MOLECULE

Strassman's project was a contribution to understanding the endogenous role in humans of DMT and its functional analogues. From the mid-1950s, a series of discoveries demonstrated that DMT and its close relatives 5-hydroxy-DMT (bufotenine) and 5-methoxy-DMT (5-MeO-DMT), are compounds naturally occurring in humans and other mammals, as detected in urine, blood, and cerebrospinal fluids.[3] With growing evidence of DMT's endogenous activity, it was observed that DMT may function as a neurotransmitter or neuromodulator.[4] Other researchers speculated that DMT may be involved in the production of dream visions.[5] That DMT was among the select compounds admitted passage across the blood-brain barrier spurred Strassman's imagination as to its purpose. Not least of all, he was driven by the awareness that precursors and enzymes necessary for DMT synthesis occur in the pineal.

Impressed by this catalogue of discoveries, Strassman was nevertheless dissatisfied with prevailing research prerogatives, largely restricted to evaluating DMT's function as a possible cause of psychoses. The limited research undertaken before federal and international interdictions took effect determined no significant differences in the levels of endogenous DMT in the body fluids of normal volunteers and those with psychotic illnesses, a result prompting science to blanche, effecting a research lacuna that would show little sign of improvement in the wake of the Controlled Substances Act of 1970. As a result of this inactivity, psychiatry was said to have 'lost a unique opportunity to probe deeper into the mysteries of consciousness'.[6] Consequently, upon prohibition and the discouragement of research, DMT would suffer a fate perhaps even more tragic than that befalling LSD. Confronting this situation, Strassman worked against the grain to consider the possibility that 'the body synthesized a compound with psychedelic properties that produced highly prized spiritual experiences, rather than highly maladaptive psychotic episodes'.[7]

This reveals what Strassman identified as the 'deeper reasons' for his investigation of DMT: 'an interest in the biological bases of naturally occurring psychedelic experiences, such as mystical and near-death states.'[8] He had been inspired by the work of Terence McKenna, who throughout the 1980s toured North America lecturing on, among other subjects, the significance of DMT's natural occurrence in humans. Attention to the spiritual merits of psychedelics is also indebted to Aldous Huxley. On this point, it is curious to note that, while his research was unavailable to English reading scientists like Strassman, DMT featured in German psychologist Adolf Dittrich's experiments in Zurich in the 1980s, enabling the development of a self-rating scale that served to quantitatively describe alternative states of consciousness. As Nicolas Langlitz has related, holding an assumption about a 'universal core experience identifying humankind as a spiritual species', Dittrich identified three states of consciousness that were intended to define in quantitative psychological terms what Huxley had called 'heaven', 'hell' and 'visions'.[9]

Strassman's investigations superseded previous efforts. A diligent transcriber of his volunteers' experiences, he formulated telling comparisons with near death experiences and alien abduction reports leading to further speculation testing the limits of science. Increasingly dissatisfied with biochemical and psychological models that served to explain away the experiences, reflecting upon the trials in which volunteers were frequently encountering beings that appear 'more real than real', Strassman was urged to take these occurrences seriously as phenomenological events.[10] What appeared compelling to his mind was that the effects of introduced DMT to a significant proportion of his volunteers were not dissimilar to what are universally reported as 'spiritual', 'enlightenment', or 'mystical' experiences, complete with blinding white light, timelessness, contact with omniscient beings, and the sensation of having died and been reborn. Strassman was compelled to find a new hermeneutic. Labelled the 'spirit molecule,' DMT may lead us to 'an acceptance of the coexistence of opposites, such as life and death, good and evil; a knowledge that consciousness continues after death; a deep understanding of the basic unity of all phenomena; and a sense of wisdom or love pervading all existence.'[11] If this was the effect of administered DMT, could this same compound produced endogenously be the physical media for mystical experience? Positioning a wedge into the tight opening on the Pandora's Box of consciousness, Strassman took to transcribing the infinite in the empiricist dicta of science, albeit in language suffused with a Buddhist worldview.

THE SPIRIT GLAND

As a lay member of a monastic community in Sacramento, Tibetan Buddhism had a shaping influence on Strassman's project, perhaps most importantly guiding speculation concerning the very purpose of DMT (i.e. its purported role in death-rebirth). That DMT affects a near-death experience was intuited from a telling synchronicity that bridged Strassman's spiritual and medical science training. He'd learned that the forty-nine days transit in which the soul reincarnates— as taught in *The Tibetan Book of the Dead*—is exactly the interval from conception to the first signs of pineal formation in the human embryo, and nearly exactly the same moment that the foetus' gender can be determined. This understanding triggered speculations concerning the hidden role of the pineal gland—what René Descartes called 'the seat of the soul'—in death and rebirth.

It seemed less hypothesis than conviction that Strassman's 'spirit gland' was 'the intermediary between the physical and the spiritual'.[12] With the proposition that the organ excretes large quantities of DMT at the moments of birth and death, the pineal is reckoned to be the 'lightning rod of the soul'. The tiny organ's central position in the epithalamus, between the two hemispheres, could allow DMT synthesised in the pineal to be secreted directly into the cerebrospinal fluid and affect visual and auditory pathways. When we die (or indeed have near-death experiences), it was supposed, 'the life force leaves the body through the pineal gland', where a DMT release is speculated to be like the floodwaters carrying the soul into the liminal phase (or bardo) between life and life, as depicted in *The Tibetan Book of the Dead.* And functioning as a kind of spirit antenna, 'pineal DMT release at forty-nine days after conception marks the entrance of the spirit into the fetus'. Although the burden of proof remains, Strassman conjectured that 'pineal tissue in the dying or recently dead may produce DMT for a few hours, and perhaps longer, and could affect our lingering consciousness. While our "dead" brain wave readings are "flat," who knows about our inner mental state at this time.'[13] The proposal that the soul is released at death from the region of the pineal is indeed depicted in Alex Grey's painting 'Dying', reproduced on the cover of Strassman's book, a painting depicting a deceased human with vapor rising from the crown, all overseen by a spiralling pattern of multiple disembodied wide-open eyes.

The pineal gland possesses vital functionality recognised by science. It regulates the hormone melatonin, which it converts from serotonin, with a balanced melatonin cycle essential for sleep, reproduction, motor activity, blood pressure, the immune system, cellular growth, and body temperature, among other vital functions. While Strassman's early research had investigated the role of melatonin in depression, it seemed depressing for a man who intuited the hidden function and purpose of the pineal that the more critical questions weren't being asked. If the pineal gland was found to secrete DMT at certain times, couldn't its proximity to crucial sensory relay stations in the brain 'explain the highly visual and auditory nature of many mystical and other endogenous psychedelic experiences'?[14] Interest in the 'psychedelic pineal gland' was evident in 1986 when Strassman was invited to speak at Esalen, meeting McKenna and Rupert Sheldrake. The hidden function of the pineal was hypothesised in a 1991 issue of *Psychedelic Monographs and Essays*, where, alongside a discussion of its role in converting melatonin from serotonin, Strassman proposed that the tiny endocrine gland in the vertebrate brain had a secret psychedelic function. Drawing inspiration from Descartes' meditations on this pinecone shaped non-paired organ's role as a conduit for the soul, he proposed that the pineal 'mediates the psychophysiological actions of what might be referred to as the consciousness-bearing life force of an individual'. Amidst detailed speculation on the mechanisms by which endogenous psychoactive tryptamines may be synthesised in the pineal, Strassman introduced his metaphysical hunch regarding the forty-nine day embryonic pineal formation coinciding with the reincarnation of the life-force according to the Thodol Bardo.[15] It soon became an underground truism that, as D.M. Turner wrote in *The Essential Psychedelics Guide*, 'DMT is produced in the human pineal gland which is correlated to the "3rd eye" or Ajna Chakra in the Indian spiritual system'. By meditating, yogis could, for instance, increase their DMT levels.[16]

News of the psychedelic function of the pineal provided an update on a gland that has exerted a magnetic influence on esotericists who've long extolled its spiritual and paranormal propensities; in particular the pineal's capacity, once activated, to enable previously dormant powers of perception, especially those associated with vision: clairvoyance, seeing auras, and being awakened to information from other dimensions. Within the esoteric milieu, the visionary capacity of the pineal has been elucidated via interwoven trajectories. The all-seeing-eye can be traced to the ancient Egyptian symbol of the Eye of Horus, recognised among occult historians as a precise graphic depiction of a cross-section of the pineal gland. The light-transducing ability of the pineal gland has led to its reception as the 'third eye,' whose activation unleashes extrasensory powers, an idea traced to Hindu traditions from which practices of meditation and Yoga have derived, and through which the activation of the crown chakra is thought to activate psychic powers. Strassman's research quickly proved important among those seeking neurochemical explanations for such extra-sensory abilities and psi-phenomena.[17]

As the pineal's latest champion, Strassman's speculations were readily absorbed within an occult science milieu where the spiritual function of the pineal was a foregone conclusion, now enjoying the support of a formal scientific investigation. 'A resonance process may occur in the pineal similar to that of shattering glass,' wrote Strassman. 'The pineal begins to 'vibrate' at frequencies that weaken its multiple barriers to DMT formation: the pineal cellular shield, enzyme levels, and quantities of anti-DMT. The end result is a psychedelic surge of the pineal spirit molecule, resulting in the subjective states of mystical consciousness.'[18] Such artful speculation met with approval among those seeking to hitch a ride on the coat-tails of science, a practice evident throughout modern esoteric thought stretching back to the Theosophists and beyond. If Helena Blavatsky had popularised the idea that an actual 'third eye' belonging to the ancients had atrophied through the course of evolution into the pineal—a faint reminder of 'the early spiritual and purely psychic characteristics in man'[19]—contemporary esotericists celebrate the means by which, like an opened third eye, the re/activation of the pineal gland enables lucid dreaming, out-of-body experiences, hypnagogic imagery, near-death experiences, astral travel, and ultimately, as Anthony Peake conveys in *The Infinite Mindfield*, the evolution of consciousness.[20] These ideas are also an echo of Blavatsky, who observed that the pineal is the key to higher consciousness. 'This seemingly useless appendage is the pendulum which, once the clock-work of the *inner* man is wound up, carries the spiritual vision of the EGO to the highest planes of perception, where the horizon open before it becomes almost infinite.'[21]

The breaking news on endogenous DMT becomes a golden arrow in the quiver of spiritual warriors like 'Hippie Jedi' and 'Freedom-Preneur' Justin Verrengia, who is on a mission to change the world one person (and one sale) at a time. Through practice and development, Verrengia claims that pineal activation can produce natural DMT allowing individuals to access 'extrasensory superpowers you never knew existed'. Psychic abilities like astral travel, exploring other dimensions, and even foreseeing the future, are at your fingertips. Moreover, when the pineal is fully operational, the individual can be, or so Verrengia ostentates, 'in a constant visionary state most of the time'. For writer and hypnotherapist Iona Miller, implicated in the production of DMT, the 'master gland' is responsible for 'the internal perception of Light, the raising of Kundalini the serpent power, and for awakening inner sight or in-sight'.

At a time when life coaches promote meditation, yoga, qigong, tai chi, and other practices to activate the brain's 'spiritual gateway' and open up 'the line of communication with the higher planes', when wellness instructors endorse dietary supplements—like neem and organic blue ice skate fish oil—that will decalcify your pineal gland and enable you to 'exploit your full spiritual capabilities',[22] where 'solar gazing' is reckoned to be an ancient activity converting solar energy into physical nourishment by way of the light-sensitive pineal,[23] where Dark Room techniques have been developed to stimulate the production of 'Pineal Soma and DMT' or 'Endohuasca',[24] or where the N3 Lucia Hypnagogic Light Machine is conjectured to stimulate DMT release, Strassman's ideas flow like quicksilver. With mounting speculation concerning the role of DMT and the pineal, those seeking to maximise their human potential and ability to access transpersonal states of consciousness could ostensibly activate, or reactivate, their third eye, through life practices designed to optimise the pineal and ensure DMT synthesis or release. Included among these life practices is the art of taking DMT.

∞∞∞∞∞∞

Strassman's chief hypothesis, that 'outside-administered DMT elicits altered states of consciousness similar to those that people report during spontaneous psychedelic experiences: near-death and mystical states and the phenomenon we call alien abduction'[25]—an overlap supporting a role for endogenous DMT release in these experiences—has fired the imagination, not only of esotericists and occult scientists, but film-makers, novelists, musicians and visionary artists. As documented in *Mystery School in Hyperspace*, with his speculations solidifying as folk knowledge, Strassman's propositions have left the clinic to possess a life of their own. That book also investigates the contested status of the pineal gland. The threshold separating the material from the spirit world, the biological interface secreting the soul from the body and even enabling the living to contact the dead, the pineal has been evaluated, circumscribed, and defended in accordance with a variety of intellectual, spiritual, and theological perspectives, each making claims over its terrain. For instance, while colleagues of Strassman, looking to the historical record of religious epiphanies, contact experiences and mystical states, contend that the pineal can produce tryptamine in DMT-flash concentrations, Andrew Gallimore speculates on DMT as an 'ancestral neuromodulator' and the possibility that the pineal gland may well have produced DMT in psychedelic quantities in the remote past.[26] With a genealogy traceable to William James, Strassman clarifies his position in his recent *DMT and the Soul of Prophecy*. The compelling comparisons between events resulting from the modern administration of DMT and those experiences native to humanity throughout history have triggered a research model counterposed to the prevailing model of neurotheology, which proposes that the brain *generates* spiritual experience, or did so in the remote past. Instead, 'theoneurology' asserts that 'the brain is the agent through which God communicates with humans'.[27]

So what are we to make of the pineal gland and its role as a bridge between spirit and matter—a role updated in the ostensible 'DMT gland'? A 2013 report that DMT was found in the pineal gland microdialysate of rats came closer to confirming Strassman's proposition.[28] And yet, even if it were confirmed that the human pineal gland produces DMT in 'hallucinogenic' quantities, what then? It would be fanciful to conclude that such a confirmation would lead to universal acceptance of Strassman's metaphysical claims regarding the spiritual function of the pineal/DMT. It is more reasonable to assume that the usual suspects will rally to entrenched positions on the nature of consciousness. But then, Strassman's ideas have gained popular appeal. While the outcomes are unpredictable, it appears that we are in the preliminary phase of a significant debate. It is difficult to ignore the theological implications of this unique research, for while his own approach—i.e. his science and indeed his faith—would be altered subsequent to the UNM project, Strassman's legacy is to have made the inquiry on DMT an investigation into the human nature of spirituality.

References:

1. Thompson, H.S, *Fear and Loathing in Las Vegas: A Savage Journey to the Heart of the American Dream*. Random House. 1971. 46.

2. For exposition of the cultural history of DMT, 'hyperspace,' and the 'breakthrough' experience, see St John, G., *Mystery School in Hyperspace: A Cultural History of DMT*. Berkeley: North Atlantic Books/Evolver. 2015. For investigation of DMT ontology, see Gallimore, A. and Luke, D. 'DMT Research from 1956 to the End of Time.' In King, D., Luke, D., Sessa, B., Adams, C., Tollan, A. (eds), *Neurotransmissions: Essays on Psychedelics from Breaking Convention*. London: Strange Attractor. 2015. 291–316. For DMT entities, see Luke, D. 2008, 'Disembodied Eyes Revisited. An Investigation into the Ontology of Entheogenic Entity Encounters.' *Entheogen Review: The Journal of Unauthorized Research on Visionary Plants and Drugs*. 2008 17(1):1–9 & 38–40.; Luke, D. 'Discarnate Entities and Dimethyltryptamine (DMT): Psychopharmacology, Phenomenology and Ontology.' *Journal of the Society for Psychical Research*. 2011 75(1):26–42.

3. For a review of this research see Barker, S.A., McIlhenny, E.H., Strassman, R. 'A Critical Review of Reports of Endogenous Psychedelic N, N-Dimethyltryptamines in Humans, 1955–2010,' *Drug Test Analysis*. 2012 4:617–635. This review suggests that compelling mass spectral evidence exists confirming the presence of DMT and its close relatives in certain human biological fluids.

4. Barker, S.A., Monti, J.A., Christian S.T., 'N, N-Dimethyltryptamine: An Endogenous Hallucinogen,' *International Review of Neurobiology*. 1981 22:83–110.

5. Callaway, J.C. 'A Proposed Mechanism for the Visions of Dream Sleep.' *Medical Hypotheses*. 1988 26(2):119–124.

6. Strassman, R. DMT, *The Spirit Molecule: A Doctor's Revolutionary Research into the Biology of Near-Death and Mystical Experiences*. Rochester, VT: Park Street Press. 2001. 49.

7. Strassman, R. *DMT and the Soul of Prophecy: A New Science of Spiritual Revelation in the Hebrew Bible*. VT: Park Street Press. 2014. 30.

8. Strassman, R. 'DMT: The Brain's Own Psychedelic.' In Strassman, R., Wojtowicz, S., Luna, L.E., Frecska, E. *Inner Paths to Outer Space: Journeys to Alien Worlds through Psychedelics and Other Spiritual Technologies*. Rochester, VT: Park Street Press. 2008. 42.

9. Langlitz, N. *Neuropsychedelia: The Revival of Hallucinogen Research Since the Decade of the Brain*. Berkeley, CA: University of California Press. 2013. 101. Franz Vollenweider later used functional neuroimaging to capture neurobiologically the states measured psychologically by Dittrich—although, as Langlitz observes, Vollenweider's research would 'support the revival of the hallucinogenic model of psychosis' (102–103).

10. Strassman, DMT: *The Spirit Molecule*, ibid. 313.

11. Ibid. 54.

12. Ibid. 60.

13. Ibid. xvii, 76.

14. Strassman, 'DMT: The Brain's Own Psychedelic,' ibid. 40.

15. Strassman, R.J. 'The Pineal Gland: Current Evidence for its Role in Consciousness'. *Psychedelic Monographs and Essays*. 1991 5 167–205. [188, 182].

16. Turner, D.M. *The Essential Psychedelics Guide.* 1994. 67.

17. For a comprehensive review of research investigating the pineal as a possible site for the production of DMT, 5-Me0-DMT and bufotinine, see Luke, D. 'Psychoactive Substances and Paranormal Phenomena: A Comprehensive Review'. *International Journal of Transpersonal Studies.* 2012 31:97–156.

18. Strassman, DMT: *The Spirit Molecule*, ibid. 75.

19. Blavatsky, H.P. *The Secret Doctrine: The Synthesis of Science, Religion and Philosophy.* Vol. II (*Anthropogenesis*). London: Theosophical Publishing Company, Ltd. 1888. 267.

20. Anthony Peake, 2013, The Infinite Mindfield: The Quest to Find the Gateway to Higher Consciousness.

21. Blavatsky, H.P. 'Dialogue on the Mysteries of the After Life [Part 2]'. *Lucifer.* Vol 3 (January 15 1889) 407–417.

22. Hunt, A. 'Top 8 Supplements to Boost Your Pineal Gland Function'. *Waking Times* (September 5 2013). http://www.wakingtimes.com/2013/09/05/top-8-supplements-boost-pinealgland-function/

23. Olsen, *Modern Esoteric*, ibid. 285.

24. Kimah, 'Interview with Ananda on Dark Room Retreat Alchemy.' http://www.akasha.de/~aton/DR.html

25. Strassman, *DMT: The Spirit Molecule*, 154.

26. Strassman, R., with Wojtowicz, S., Luna, L.E., Frecska, E. *Inner Paths to Outer Space: Journeys to Alien Worlds through Psychedelics and Other Spiritual Technologies.* Rochester, VT: Park Street Press. 2008. Gallimore, A.R. 'Building Alien Worlds—The Neuropsychological and Evolutionary Implications of the Astonishing Psychoactive Effects of N,N-Dimethyltryptamine (DMT)'. *Journal of Scientific Exploration* 2013 27, no. 3: 455–503.

27. Strassman, *DMT and the Soul of Prophecy*, ibid. 4.

28. Barker, S.A., Borjigin. J., Lomnicka, I., Strassman, R. 'LC/MS/MS Analysis of the Endogenous Dimethyltryptamine Hallucinogens, Their Precursors, and Major Metabolites in Rat Pineal Gland Microdialysate.' *Biomedical Chromatography* 2013 27, no. 12: 1690–1700.

ON VISION AND BEING HUMAN: TOWARDS A MORE HOLISTIC IMAGE

BRUCE RIMELL

As an artist who works with the visionary, the dreamlike, the sacred and the archetypal, it might seem reasonable to assume that I am acutely concerned with the question: what is Visionary Art? Strange as it is to say, I am not very concerned with this question, being happy enough to suggest that Visionary Art is simply what it says: the art of visions, of dreams, of sacred journeys inwards and meditative insights, among many other things.[1] It is the phenomena that this artform seeks to depict that interest me, rather than the artform itself, and really we are just delaying the question.

What, then, is a vision? If my art is a vehicle for anything, it is to answer this question, in as many different ways as I am able. This problem has also occupied my thinking for a great deal of time, and like many quintessentially human phenomena, it is much easier to list its properties than to give a solid definition free from metaphor or analogy with other human experiences or behaviours. One of the principle properties of visionary and religious experiences is that they appear to provide an experiential or evidential report from a hidden reality, a sensation that Rudolf Otto termed 'wholly other'[2] and as a condition 'absolutely *sui generis* and incomparable [to everyday reality] whereby the human being finds himself utterly abashed'.[3]

Those of us who regularly experience visions—whether entheogenically-inspired, spontaneously emergent or driven by trance based ritual, or through migraines and other neurological glitches[4]—may recognise the territory. This hidden reality has many names: the Platonic World of Forms,[5] the Ultimate Ground of Being,[6] the Kingdom of God or of Heaven,[7] the World Beyond Worlds.[8] It is wholly unlike the 'real' world: indeed it is often hyper-real, more real and more intense than anything in our everyday reality.[9] It is infused with an immanent supernatural power, it shimmers with animism, light and presence whereby every action, event and moment is suffused with meaning and intentionality.[10] It shapeshifts, so that deities fuse with archetypes, and externalised mythical images become embodied in the visionary subject.

These attributes of 'otherness' or of coming from a hidden reality, of animism, of supernatural power and intentionality, are ubiquitous enough in visionary narratives to constitute essential aspects, but considering everything that we know in the 21st century, each one of them is problematic in one form or another.

For example, quantum mechanics informs us that such a hidden reality cannot possibly exist.[11] In stark contrast to the popular view of QM as being dependent on consciousness and subjectivity, or that a loosely-termed 'Uncertainty Principle' means that what one observes one changes, the mathematical structure and experimental observation of QM actually demonstrates something much more unsettling for the human psyche. There is an objective reality, a 'real' world of the everyday, but this objectivity is not fundamental. Rather it is emergent,[12] a surface feature arising out of a morass of quantum interactions founded ultimately upon indeterminacy, a lack of realism and no *a priori* foundational characteristic.[13] There is a void under reality, and its nature is absent (Rimell, 2015, p49), a situation not well-suited to the perception of an external hidden reality seen by the visionary senses.

Modern evidential enquiry has also found no sign of deity, nor do we see any sense that the universe contains a supernatural power of the type ubiquitous in human understanding: neither *shakti* nor *kundalini*, neither *n/um* nor *mana* has presented itself to objective scientific discourse. What, then, is to be done with this situation, which is a significant problem for modern humanity? In the past century or so, two dominant paradigms have presented themselves as the solution to the issue.

The first is dismissal: visionary experience, along with deities and all notions of supernatural power, animism and intentionality are to be rejected as irrational, meaningless, generally delusional, and moreover anathema to proper science.[14] This approach is not actually that modern: in Western culture for at least 2,500 years, humanity's primary cultural responsibility has not been to eternity or the primordial repetition of exemplary mythical gestures, but to history and to actions and events within that history.[15] In this view, to engage with vision is to lose oneself in fantasy. This is a most unsatisfactory response to these experiences, and somewhat ironically closes off a great many important scientific and introspective questions to our purview.

The second paradigm is a kind of literalism: the individual contents of visions might be local to a culture or particular to an individual, but basic visionary properties are considered as absolutely real, that they really do represent evidential reports from a literal hidden reality, that supernatural power is actual but inexplicably non-material, events of the world really are guided by a transcendent intentionality often personified as deity.[16] This is equally unsatisfying, and can only thrive in a world where certain scientific insights are either misunderstood or excised from view, or where a realm of confused pseudo-science or religious nostalgia holds sway, neither of which are particularly authentic to the colourful experience of visionary mindstates, nor do they disclose in my view much in the way of truth about our humanity.

There seems to me to be no meaningful compromise readily available for these opposing views, and much of popular discourse in the modern West appears to venerate the notion of picking a side and fighting one's corner rather than seeking common ground.[17] One possible solution to this conundrum need not take the shape of such compromise, but rather that the study and wider acceptance of the intrinsic value of visionary experience requires new information to effect a transcending of the issue, getting past a bivalent oppositional mentality towards something deeper and more fundamental to both science and vision.

There is one facet of human behaviour which I believe has precisely this property: symbolic cognition.[18]

An insight from palaeoanthropology and evolutionary psychology is that, as soon as humans arrive on the scene, we seem to surround ourselves with non-functional objects: handaxes which are much too large to be useful[19] and a rising obsession with red ochre, a substance with little to no practical function.[20] At length, we began to create geometric designs,[21] and handprints on rock walls as one of the earliest artforms appears to express a desire to be intimate with something unseen.[22]

Symbolic culture has been termed as 'an environment of objective facts whose existence depends entirely on subjective belief',[23] a 'communal map'[24] or unseen world of reference[25] through which individualist perceptions and cognitions are altered in favour of collective motivations. It is this collective unreality, through which human behaviour operates, that forms our hallmark attribute. Both automatic and volitional,[26] symbolic cognition is what separates us not just from animals, but from previous species of human too.

It appears to be founded principally upon the pre-frontal cortex, which is highly developed in cognitively-modern humans. This cortex mediates 'our ability to plan, conceptualise, symbolise... and form abstract ideas. It also controls physiological drives and turns basic feelings into complex emotions...'[27] and despite being only very recently evolved, it appears to have sent out connections all across the brain to favour a kind of top-down processing[28] in which these symbolic functions are allowed to dominate our cognition.

This top-down approach is seen not just in the individual but in society too. One way in which symbolic culture and constructs are reified is through ritual and collective action, which is costly and demonstrates commitment to the group, suppressing individual desires.[29] This generates trust,[30] which is essential for symbolic culture to flourish, as engagement with fictional constructs and counter-reality cannot operate in an environment where the egotistical and Machiavellian drives typical of great apes predominate.[31] Early human ritual actions may have included dance or ecstatic movements that could function ambiguously as both sexually selective display—perceptually verifiable realities of fitness—and symbolic drama—enacting unseen worlds—and here we may find a possible origin for visionary experience, in the trance states engendered by repetitive movements.[32]

Crucially, while symbolic culture and cognition is largely based upon human social and neurological realities, from a subjective point of view visionary and religious experience makes the unseen world of symbolic reference visible and available to direct experience.[33] This begins to effect a kind of visionary 'virtuous circle' in human behaviour.

There are fine-grained models within evolutionary psychology that can elucidate why our propensity for symbolic cognition is adaptive.[34] These models are complex, but it appears that this counter-intuitive piece of our cognitive architecture could be sexually selective, and there is within human female reproductive behaviour a powerful analogical complement to the 'unseen world of symbolic reference', or the expectation of a hidden reality, and this is menstruation.

From a signalling perspective, menstruation combined with a complete suppression of all other fertility signals is an unusual behaviour for a flexibly intelligent primate,[35] but if we consider that symbols are made real through ritual, and visions make hidden worlds visible, then menstruation can be said to make an unseen fertility visible.[36] Amplification of this menstrual signal through ritual action and body painting may explain the perennial early human obsession with red ochre.[37] This is an oversimplified analogy of the problem, but we are suddenly gazing at a much wider image of the human being than a limited purview of visionary experience, of trance or of religious insights might lead us to expect. These models can also explicate the emergence of humanity's first deities, as red-ochre painted dancers[38] embodying an unseen symbolic system.

What does all this mean for us in the 21st century? I have only briefly listed some relevant points rather than explored them in detail, but we can see that collective unrealities and expectations of hidden worlds appear to be delocalised across the whole human being— sexual selection, ritual behaviour, menstruation, social realities, neurology and cognition all contain aspects of this uniquely human phenomenon.[39] The enfolding of 'unseen worlds of reference' can also be seen in the deep structure of language, and the drive to express them in artistic, embodied and dramatic form is as ubiquitous a human behaviour as the visionary and religious experiences they depict.

Contrary to what we may be led to believe from the sensations delivered to our perception, visionary experience does not provide an evidential report into a literal hidden reality, but that does not necessitate a strict cult of reason in which it must be dismissed as unreal or irrational.[40] Indeed in its attachment to both abstraction and symbol,[41] the pre-frontal cortex appears to transcend the modern artificial boundary of reason and unreason, since both the scientific method and the visionary approach to living both deeply benefit from its actions and propensities.[42] Symbolic cognition is both the method by which scientific theses are formulated, and the driving force behind the pervasive sense of meaning and intentionality in visionary experience.

Unreality operates at every level of the human being, and if in the 21st century we are to come to terms with ourselves holistically and with genuine wellness of a unified mind and body, these subjectively-collective fictions—gods, the experience of supernatural potency and visionary animisms—need to be integrated into our self-understanding. Anything else is setting ourselves against our own human nature. Visionary artists are well-placed to effect this kind of integration, in a realm where fact and non-fact, or belief and non-belief, are less useful than dynamics of relevance, of experience, of imagination, and of creativity. Humans are flexibly intelligent,[43] and visionary experience emerging from a ubiquitous propensity for symbolic cognition is crucial to this flexibility.

My rising feeling over the past few years has been that we are now in a position to transcend limiting ideas which spring from projected literalisms or cynical dismissals, towards an inwardly-focussed humanism in which we creatively centre all these magical hidden worlds, unrealities and shimmering animisms upon ourselves and our wonderfully complex evolved minds, and hence to begin a movement away from visionary 'otherness' to a kind of 'sacred intimacy'—hidden worlds within us—in which we can delight in a deeper and more holistic image of an evidentially-enquiring, symbolically-perceiving, materialistic-but-otherworldly, paradoxical-and-experiential sacred human being.

References

1. Caruana, 2001, p35 & pp37–48.

2. Otto, 1923 in Eliade, 1987 pp9–10.

3. Otto, 1923, p7 & p45.

4. Rimell, 2014, passim.

5. Buckingham et al., 2011, pp50–55.

6. Grey, 2015, passim.

7. Davies, 2002, pp137–39.

8. Rimell, 2015, pp28–33.

9. Rimell, 2015, p30.

10. Campbell, 1990, p48.

11. Bell, 1964, passim; Kirchmair et al., 2009, passim; Mermin, 1985, p3; Griffiths, 1998, p423.

12. Dirac, 1933, passim.

13. Siegel, 2014, passim; Susi, 2015, personal communication; summarised in Rimell, 2015 pp45–47.

14. for example Dawkins, 2007, p188; Atran, 2002, viii; see also Rimell, 2015, p228-30 & p279–80.

15. Eliade, 1989, passim.

16. for example Strassman, 2001, pp316-18; Rimell, 2015, pp184–5; see also Lewis-Williams, 2002, p129.

17. Rimell, 2015, pp163–72.

18. de Lumley, 2009, p10; Knight, Power & Watts, 1995, p77; Chase, 1994, p628; Rimell, 2015, pp83–86.

19. Kohn & Mithen, 1999, passim.

20. Watts, 2002, passim; Knight, Power & Watts, pp85–87.

21. Saura Ramos, 1998, pp32–4.

22. Rimell, 2016, passim.

23. Knight, 2010, p193.

24. Knight, Power & Watts, 1995, p77.

25. Rimell, 2015, p23.

26. Rimell, 2015, p67; see also Kohn, 1999, p249 & Mithen, 1996, p179 & pp185–194 on cognitive fluidity.

27. Lent, 2010, p1.

28. van Slyke, 2011, p113: see also Dietrich, 2003, pp232–5.

29. Knight, 1991, p80; Power, 2001, pp20–26.

30. Watts, 2009, p92.

31. Knight, 2010, passim; see also Knight, Power & Watts, 1995, p76.

32. Rimell, 2015, pp107–9 & pp112–13.

33. Rimell, 2015, p113 & pp160–61.

34. Knight, 1991, passim; Knight, Power & watts, 1995, passim; Power, 2001, passim.

35. Knight, Power & Watts, 1995, p78; Kohn, 1999, pp199–200.

36. Power, 2001, p134.

37. Power, 2001, pp134–42 & pp180-84; see also Rimell, 2015, pp87–93.

38. Power, 2001, p163; see also Rimell, 2015, pp107–09.

39. Rimell, 2015, pp159–62.

40. Rimell, 2015, pp165–66 & pp271–72, note 12.

41. Lent, 2010, p1.

42. Rimell, 2015, p166.

43. Kohn, 1999, p249.

Sources:

Atran, S. *In Gods We Trust: The Evolutionary Landscape of Religion*. Oxford University Press. 2002.

Bell, J.S. 'On the Einstein-Podolsky-Rosen Paradox, 1964'. Physics 1:3, http://www.drchinese.com/David/Bell_Compact.pdf, retrieved June 2014.

Buckingham, W., King, P.J., Burnham, D., Weeks, M., Hill, C., Marenbon, J. et al. *The Philosophy Book*. Dorling Kindersley. 2011.

Campbell, J. 'Bios and Mythos'. In Campbell, J. *The Flight of the Wild Gander: Explorations in the Mythological Dimensions of Fairy Tales, Legends and Symbols*. Harper Perennial. 1990.

Caruana, L. *First Draft of A Manifesto of Visionary Art*. Recluse Publishing. 2001.

Chase, P.G. 'On Symbols and the Palaeolithic'. *Current Anthropology*. 1994 35:5.

Davies, S. *The Gospel of Thomas: Annotated and Explained*. Darton, Longman & Todd. 2002.

Dawkins, R. *The God Delusion*. Black Swan. 2007.

de Lumley, H. 'The Emergence of Symbolic Thought: The Principle Steps of Hominisation Leading Towards Greater Complexity'. In *Becoming Human: Innovation in Prehistoric Material and Spiritual Culture*. Renfrew, C., Morley, I. (eds). Cambridge University Press. 2009.

Dietrich, A. 'Functional neuroanatomy of altered states of consciousness: The transient hypofrontality hypothesis'. *Consciousness and Cognition*. 2003 12.

Dirac, P.A.M. 'The Lagrangian in quantum mechanics'. *Physikalische Zeitschrift der Sowjetunion*. 1933 3. http://www.ifi.unicamp.br/~cabrera/teaching/aula%2015%202010s1.pdf, retrieved January 2015.

Eliade, M. *The Sacred and the Profane: The Nature of Religion*. Trask, W.R (trans). Harcourt Inc. 1987.

Eliade, M. *The Myth of the Eternal Return: Cosmos and History* Trask, W.R (trans). Penguin Arkana. 1989.

Grey, A. 'Cosmic Philosophy'. On Alex Grey, dated January 2015. http://alexgrey.com/cosmic-philosophy/, retrieved February 2015.

Griffiths, David J. *Introduction to Quantum Mechanics*. Pearson/Prentice Hall. 1998.

Kirchmair, G., Zähringer, F., Gerritsma, R., Kleinmann, M., Gühne, O., Cabello, A., Blatt, R., Roos, C.F. 'State-independent Experimental Test of Quantum Contextuality'. *Nature*. 2009 460, http://arxiv.org/abs/0904.1655, retrieved July 2014.

Knight, C. *Blood Relations: Menstruation and the Origins of Culture*. Yale University Press. 1991.

Knight, C. 'The Origins of Symbolic Culture'. In *Homo Novus—A Human Without Illusions*. Frey, U.J, Störmer, C., Willführ, K.P. (eds). Springer-Verlag. 2010.

Knight, C., Power, C., Watts, I. 'The Human Symbolic Revolution: A Darwinian Account'. *Cambridge Archaeological Journal*. 1995 5.

Kohn, M. *As We Know It: Coming to Terms with an Evolved Mind*. Granta Publications. 1999.

Kohn, M., Mithen, S. 'Handaxes: Products of Sexual Selection?' *Antiquity* 1999 73.

Lent, J. 'Tyranny of the Pre-Frontal Cortex'. Draft chapter of book variously titled *Finding the Li: Towards a Democracy of Consciousnes*s or *The Patterning Instinct: A Cognitive History of Humanity's Search for Meaning*, dated 2010. https://jeremylent.files.wordpress.com/2010/07/chapter-1_the-tyranny-of-the-prefrontal-cortex1.pdf, retrieved September 2014.

Lewis-Williams, D. *The Mind In The Cave: Consciousness and the Origins of Art*. Thames & Hudson. 2002.

Mermin, N.D. 'Is the moon there when nobody looks? Reality and the quantum theory'. *Physics Today*. April 1985. http://www.physics.smu.edu/scalise/EPR/References/mermin_moon.pdf, retrieved January 2015.

Mithen, S. *The Prehistory of the Mind: The Cognitive Origins of Art and Science*. Thames & Hudson. 1996.

Otto, R. *The Idea of the Holy: An Inquiry into the Non-Rational Factor in the Idea of the Divine and its Relation to the Rational.* Harvey, J.W. (trans). Oxford University Press. 1923.

Power, C. *Beauty Magic: Deceptive Sexual Signalling and the Evolution of Ritual.* Unpublished thesis, University College London. 2001. http://www.radicalanthropologygroup.org/old/pub_power_phd.pdf, retrieved June 2014.

Rimell, B. 'The Migraine as Archaic Visionary Experience'. On Archaic Visions, 2014 (ii). http: //www.visionaryartexhibition.com/archaic-visions /the-migraine-as-archaic-visionary-experience, retrieved August 2014.

Rimell, B. *On Vision and Being Human: Exploring the Menstrual, Neurological and Symbolic Origins of Religious Experience.* Xibalba Books. 2015.

Rimell, B. *Liminal Contact: A Cognitive and Anthropological Response to the 'Death' of Painting.* Xibalba Books. 2016 (forthcoming).

Saura Ramos, P.A. *The Cave of Altamira.* Harry N. Abrams, Inc. 1998.

Siegel, E. 'What is a Quantum Observation?' on Starts With A Bang, dated July 2014. http://medium.com/starts-with-a-bang/ask-ethan-46-what-is-a-quantum-observation-57d2940175e1, retrieved February 2015.

Strassman, R. *DMT—The Spirit Molecule: A Doctor's Revolutionary Research into the Biology of Near-Death and Mystical Experiences.* Park Street Press. 2001.

Susi, T. Personal communication regarding quantum observations. February 2015.

van Slyke, J.A. *The Cognitive Science of Religion.* Ashgate Science and Religion Series, Ashgate Publishing. 2011.

Watts, I. 'Ochre in the Middle Stone Age of Southern Africa: Ritualised Display or Hide Preservative?' *The South African Archaeological Bulletin.* 2002. Vol. 57, no. 175, 1–14.

Watts, I. 'Red Ochre, Body Painting, and Language: Interpreting the Blombos Ochre'. In *The Cradle of Language.* Botha, R., Knight, C. (eds). Oxford University Press. 2009.

SUBJECTIVE EFFECTS OF HOLOTROPIC BREATHWORK AND PSYCHEDELICS: A COMPARISON

IKER PUENTE

During the last decades different ways to measure mystical experiences have been developed. In general, the field of mystical experience research is characterised by a lack of uniformity regarding definitions, methods and instrumentation (Lukoff and Lu, 1988). Different authors have proposed different criteria and characteristics to define this experience, including William James (1986), Evelyn Underhill (1993), W. Stace (1960), R.C. Zaehner (1961), A. Maslow (1968) and Walter Pahnke (1963, 1966), and different questionnaires have been developed to measure this experience (Hood, 1975; Pahnke, 1963). Among the most used questionnaires we can find the *Hood Mysticism Scale* (HMS) and the *States of Consciousness Questionnaire* (SCQ), both based in the characterisations of the features of mystical experiences provided by Stace (1960).

The modern empirical study of mysticism has focused on measuring the mystical experiences that individuals have had across their lifetime. The most widely used quantitative measure of lifetime mystical experiences is the *Hood Mysticism Scale* (HMS) (Hood, 1975;

Hood and Williamson, 2000), which has been shown to be a reliable and cross-culturally valid measure of lifetime experiences.

The SCQ is a modified version of the Mystical Experience Questionnaire (MEQ), also known as the Peak Experience Profile (PEP), originally developed in the 1960s by Walter Pahnke (1963, 1966) with the aim of measuring and evaluating the potential single mystical experiences occasioned by psilocybin. The MEQ was developed based on the classic descriptive work on mystical experiences and the psychology of religion by Stace (1960), and covers the main dimensions of classic mystical experience which he describes as: 1) unity (external and internal), 2) transcendence of time and space, 3) alleged ineffability, 4) paradoxicality (claim of difficulty in describing the experience in words), 5) sense of sacredness, 6) objectivity and reality (claim of intuitive knowledge of ultimate reality), 7) deeply felt positive mood, and 8) transiency.

Pahnke performed a double-blind experiment to determine if the administration of high doses of psilocybin with an appropriate environment and preparation could produce or induce mystical experiences. The author found that the participants who received psilocybin experienced more intensely the phenomenon that was described and characterised as mystical experience (Pahnke, 1963; Pahnke, 1966).

The original version of the MEQ has been modified and expanded over the years for its use in subsequent psychedelic research (Di Leo, 1982; Richards, 1975). New categories measuring transpersonal but not necessarily mystical experiences were added (Doblin, 1991). A modified version of the questionnaire, the SCQ, was developed and administered recently by Griffiths et al. (2006, 2008, 2011) to conduct a number of studies to characterise the mystical-type effects of psilocybin using double-blind and placebo controlled methodologies.

The recent studies conducted by Ronald Griffiths and William Richards' team at the Department of Neuroscience at Johns Hopkins University have replicated and extended the research conducted by Pahnke in the 1960s (Griffiths et al., 2006, 2008, 2011). Griffiths et al. (2006) conducted a double-blind study evaluating the immediate (7h) and medium-term effects (2–14 months) of a high dose of psilocybin, at a psychological level and in the state of mood, compared with an active placebo, administered in a comfortable atmosphere and with therapeutic support. Griffiths et al. found that psilocybin produced a 'complete' mystical type experience in 61% of the volunteers (in 22 of the 36 subjects who participated in the study). At 2 months, volunteers rated the experience as very significant personally and spiritually, and attributed sustained positive changes in their attitudes and behaviour. In 2008 Griffiths et al. published another article describing the persistent, long-term effects that these experiences had on volunteers, 14 months later. They concluded that, when administered in a comfortable setting and with interpersonal support, psilocybin produces mystical type experiences similar to spontaneous mystical experiences, and that these experiences were considered by the volunteers among the most personally and spiritually significant experiences of their lives 14 months after the experience.

Griffiths et al. (2011) also conducted a dose-effect study with psilocybin in 18 volunteers, using 4 different doses of the substance in 4 sessions conducted at intervals of 1 month. Griffiths et al. found that the percentage of volunteers who had a complete mystical experience increased with the dose (being 0, 5.6, 11.1, 44.4 and 55.6 for doses of 0, 5, 10, 20 and 30mg/70kg respectively). They also found that, in high doses, volunteers considered the experience with psilocybin as very significant personally and spiritually, 1 month and 14 months after the session.

Historically, the MEQ/PEP and the SCQ have been used to measure the subjective effects of psilocybin and other classic psychedelic compounds, and several studies have demonstrated the sensitivity of this questionnaire to the effects of psilocybin, LSD and other psychedelics (Pahnke, 1963, 1966; Pahnke and Richards, 1966; Richards et al., 1972, 1977). Nevertheless, it has rarely been used for the evaluation of the potential mystical experiences occasioned by other techniques employed in the context of transpersonal psychology and psychotherapy, such as Holotropic Breathwork.

Holotropic Breathwork (HB) is a technique developed and used in the context of transpersonal psychology to induce non-ordinary states of consciousness and transpersonal experiences. HB was developed in the mid-70s by Stanislav Grof, one of the founders of transpersonal psychology (Grof, 1988, 2000; Grof and Grof, 2010), after two decades working with LSD and other psychedelic substances in psychotherapy (Grof, 1972, 1975, 1980). This method was conceived as a non-drug way of accessing non-ordinary states of consciousness and transpersonal experiences. HB is a novel, experientially oriented, therapeutic technique that involves a number of diverse elements, including music, elective bodywork and accelerated breathing. HB sessions usually last between 2 and 3 hours, and are terminated voluntarily by the client. Both individual and group therapies are possible, but the group therapy context is the most commonly used.

According to Grof, the HB can induce different kinds of transpersonal experiences, including mystical experiences, among others (Grof, 1985; Grof and Grof, 2010). Grof's claims are based on more than three decades of work with this technique, and on anecdotal observations and subjective reports of many of the participants in his workshops and HB sessions.

The aim of the present study is to measure the subjective effects occasioned by HB using the SCQ, specifically looking to the occurrence of mystical experiences, and to compare them with the subjective effects produced by psilocybin.

METHOD

Participants

In this pilot study, a convenient sample was used. Eligible participants were individuals enrolled in a weeklong HB workshop held at a wellness and personal growth centre. Eligibility criteria were as follows: aged 18 to 35, English speaking, and able to provide informed consent. Both 'first breathers' (participants who were exposed to HB for first time) and those who had previous experience were allowed to take part in the research. No control group was used in the present study.

All the participants of the retreat who completed the inclusion criteria (N=49) were approached about participating in the study. From all the participants of the retreat (N=140), 29 individuals filled out the SCQ after their first HB session. Participants in the study (N=29) age ranged between 19 and 34 years (Mean=26.7, S.D.=3.94). Seventeen of the participants were female (58.6%) and 12 were male (41.4%). Fourteen participants were 'first breathers', and another 15 had previous experience with HB.

Psychometric measures/materials

The variable examined was measured with the *States of Consciousness Questionnaire* (SCQ). The SCQ is a self-assessed 100-item questionnaire, which was designed to assess mystical experiences based on the classic descriptive work on mystical experiences and the psychology of religion by Stace (1960). It provides scale scores for each of seven domains of mystical experiences: internal unity (pure awareness; a merging with ultimate reality); external unity (unity of all things; all things are alive; all is one); transcendence of time and space; ineffability and paradoxicality (claim of difficulty in describing the experience in words); sense of sacredness (awe); noetic quality (claim of intuitive knowledge of ultimate reality); and deeply felt positive mood (joy, peace, and love). The data on each scale were expressed as a proportion of the maximum possible score, fixed at 1. Based on prior research (Pahnke, 1969), the criteria for considering a volunteer as having had a 'complete' mystical experience were that the scores on each of the following scales had to be at least 0.6: unity (either internal or external, whichever was greater), transcendence of time and space, ineffability and paradoxicality, sense of sacredness, noetic quality, and deeply felt positive mood. Forty-three items on this questionnaire comprised the Pahnke–Richards MEQ/PEP (Pahnke, 1969; Richards 1975), and the remaining 57 items in the questionnaire served as distracter items.

Procedure

The data were collected after each of the two HB sessions that each participant had during the workshop. The workshop was held at a human development centre near New York in October 2009, and the researcher stayed at the centre all week to collect the data. Permission to conduct the study was requested from and granted by the organiser and the directors of the workshop. After the introductory talk of the workshop, all the participants were invited to participate in the research and to fill out a consent form, a sociodemographic survey and the SCQ questionnaire. Participants were told that the study was part of the researcher's study on HB. Participation in the study was completely voluntary. Written informed consent was obtained prior to the assessments. The questionnaire and survey took around 20–30 minutes to fill out. No compensation was offered for participation in the study.

RESULTS

Data analyses

The data were statistically analysed for the 29 volunteers who completed the SCQ using the 17.0 version of SPSS.

Measure of the *Subjective effects* of the HB
assessed during the workshop

Twenty-nine of the participants in the study filled out the SCQ after their first HB session during the workshop. Based on prior criteria, 6 volunteers had a 'complete' mystical experience during their first HB session during the workshop (20.7% of the participants who filled out the SCQ). Three of the volunteers who had a 'complete' mystical experience were 'first breathers', and the other 3 had previous experience with the HB. The higher scores of the SCQ were found on 'ineffability' (0.58), 'intuitive knowledge' (0.5) and 'deeply felt positive mood' (0.46) subscales (see Table 1).

Questionnaire	Sub-dimension	First HB session (N=29)
States of Consciousness Questionnaire	Internal Unity	0.41
	External Unity	0.33
	Transcendence of time and space	0.43
	Ineffability	0.58
	Sacredness	0.45
	Intuitive knowledge	0.5
	Deeply felt positive mood	0.46
	"Complete" mystical experience	N=6 (20.7%)

Note: Data are mean scores with the SD shown in parentheses. For the seven sub-dimensions of the States of Consciousness Questionnaire, data are expressed as a proportion of the maximum possible score, fixed at 1.

TABLE 1: Volunteers' ratings (N=29) on the States of Consciousness Questionnaire (SCQ) completed 1 to 5 hours after the first HB session.

SCQ sub-dimensions and total score	First HB session (N=29)	Psilocybin 10mg (N=18)	Psilocybin 20mg (N=18)
Internal unity	0.41	0.45	0.64
External unity	0.33	0.35	0.53
Transcendence of time and space	0.43	0.44	0.71
Ineffability	0.58	0.59	0.65
Sacredness	0.45	0.54	0.65
Noetic quality	0.5	0.54	0.68
Deeply felt positive mood	0.46	0.57	0.73
"Complete" mystical experience	N=6 (20.7%)	N=2 (11.1%)	N=6 (44.4%)

Note: For the seven sub-dimensions of the SCQ, data are expressed as a proportion of the maximum possible score, fixed at 1.

TABLE 3: Comparison between volunteers' ratings on the SCQ after their first HB sessions and the ratings for the 10mg/70kg and 20mg/70kg psilocybin doses obtained by Griffiths et al. (2011) in their dose-response study.

DISCUSSION

The purpose of the present study was to explore the subjective effects of an HB session in the context of a weeklong residential workshop, specifically looking at the occurrence of mystical experiences, and comparing them with the subjective effects occasioned by psilocybin. The overall results of this study suggest that HB, administered to healthy individuals in the context of a weeklong workshop, is capable of occasioning 'complete' mystical experiences. Thus, the study provides some initial positive findings regarding the possible usefulness of this technique to induce mystical experiences in the context of a weeklong workshop.

In the present study, 6 participants met criteria for 'complete' mystical experience in the SCQ after their first HB session (20.7% of the volunteers who filled out the SCQ). Compared with the rate of mystical experiences obtained in the different studies using high doses of psilocybin (61% found by Griffiths et al.), the percentage of participants who met criteria for 'complete' mystical experience in the SCQ is lower during HB. If we look to the percentages of mystical experiences obtained by Griffiths et al. (2011) in their dose-effect study with psilocybin (being 0, 5.6, 11.1, 44.4 and 55.6 for doses of 0, 5, 10, 20 and 30mg/70kg respectively), the percentage obtained in the present study (20.7%) and the scores in each subscale, are closer to the 10mg/70kg psilocybin dose (11.1) obtained by Griffiths et al. (see table 2), and the scores obtained in each subscale are very similar. Puente (2015) also found a similar outcome in a previous study exploring the effects of HB in the contexts of a day-long workshop in a Russian adult sample (N=134), in which 13 volunteers had a 'complete' mystical experience during their HB session (9.7% of the volunteers).

Three of the volunteers who had a 'complete' mystical experience were 'first breathers', and the other 3 had previous experience with HB. These data suggests that subjects who have no previous experience with the HB technique are not more likely to have a mystical experience.

This finding is partially consistent with previous research on the topic. Puente (2015) found a similar outcome in the study exploring the effects of HB in the contexts of a day-long workshop in a Russian adult sample (N=134), in which 8 of the 13 volunteers who had a 'complete' mystical experience were 'first breathers' (61.5%), and the other 5 had previous experience with HB (38.5%).

In the present study, the higher scores were found in the ineffability (0.58), intuitive knowledge (0.5) and deeply felt positive mood (0.46) subscales of the SCQ. The high score in the 'deeply felt positive mood' subscale (0.46) might indicate that the subjective experience during the HB session is remembered and assessed as having an overall positive tone, more than a negative one. Puente also found that the higher scores of the SCQ were obtained on 'deeply felt positive mood' (0.57) in a previous study (Puente, 2014), followed by transcendence of time and space (0.43) and internal unity (0.43).

The results obtained in the present study also support Grof´s claims of the potential of HB to induce mystical experiences (Grof, 1985). Therefore, the outcomes found in the SCQ during the HB session in the present study seem to confirm Grof´s statement of the potential of HB to induce similar experiences to those found when he was working with psychedelics (Grof and Grof, 2010). We found that HB can induce mystical experiences of the same type as those produced by psilocybin, although less frequently and in a smaller percentage of participants (Griffiths et al., 2006). Furthermore, our results indicate that the percentage of participants having mystical experiences during an HB session is similar to the percentage obtained by Griffiths et al. (2011) using a 10mg/70kg psilocybin dose (11.1%), and lower compared with the 20mg/70kg psilocybin dose (44.4%).

Despite some initial positive findings suggesting that the use of HB in the context of a weeklong workshop might induce mystical experiences, some limitations can be pointed out which are also relevant to the present study. First, a convenient sample was used for the present study, and there was no comparison group. Thus, we cannot draw cause-effect statements from it. Second, the 29 participants of the present study only represent around 20% of the total number of participants of the workshop. Thus, these results cannot be generalised to all the participants of the weeklong workshop, or to other contexts where HB is used, but they do support the idea that HB may contribute to induce mystical experiences in this specific sample.

Nevertheless, it is remarkable that HB occasioned mystical experiences in some participants during the weeklong workshop, because the present study is one of the first to measure these kinds of experiences using the SCQ during an HB session. It is also remarkable that almost 1 out of each of 5 volunteers who filled out the SCQ had a complete mystical experience (20.7%), considering the relative low frequency of these kinds of experiences in other contexts. Similar outcomes have been found in human research with psychedelic compounds like LSD and psilocybin (Grof, 2001; Griffiths et al., 2006, 2008; MacLean et al. 2011; Pahnke, 1963, 1967). Moreover, these experiences have been related to improvements in several mental health measures (Grof, 2001; Griffiths et al., 2006, 2008).

CONCLUSIONS AND FUTURE PROJECTS

Further research into the subjective effects of HB and the potential to occasion mystical experience using this technique is needed. There are a number of areas of potential interest that might be examined in future research, including: the assessment of physiological and neurophysiologic variables, and the use of qualitative methodology, to try to find correlations between them; the subjective experiences of the participants during the HB sessions as breathers and, specifically, with the occurrence of mystical experiences. We also believe that the setting, the context surrounding the experience, is very important in relation to the subjective effects that this technique can induce. Thus, future research examining the degree to which these results are specific to the context is needed. The development of similar studies in other contexts where HB and other similar hyperventilation procedures are used could be very fruitful.

Despite its limitations, and recognising the exploratory nature of this pilot study, our results show that HB occasioned mystical experiences in some of the volunteers in the context of a weeklong workshop. These preliminary results give support for further research on the subjective effects induced by this technique, as well to the study of the possible link between these subjective effects and the possible increase in wellbeing and life satisfaction of the people who report mystical experiences during the HB sessions.

Sources:

Di Leo, F. *Protocol: LSD-assisted psychotherapy correlation of peak experience profiles with behaviour change. Appendix C: Peak experience profile.* 1982. Unpublished.

Doblin, R. 'Pahnke's 'good Friday experiment': A long-term follow-up and methodological critique'. *Journal of Transpersonal Psychology.* 1991 23(1):1–28.

Griffiths, R.R., Johnson, M.W., Richards, W.A., Richards, B.D., McCann, U., Jesse, R. 'Psilocybin occasioned mystical-type experiences: immediate and persisting dose-related effects'. *Psychopharmacology.* 2011 218:649–665.

Griffiths, R.R., Richards, W.A., McCann, U., & Jesse, R. 'Psilocybin can occasion mystical-type experiences having substantial and sustained personal meaning and spiritual significance'. *Journal of Psychopharmacology.* 2006 187:268–283.

Griffiths, R.R., Richards, W.A., Johnson, M.W., McCann, U., Jesse, R. 'Mystical type experiences occasioned by psilocybin mediate the attribution of personal meaning and spiritual significance 14 months later'. *Journal of Psychopharmacology.* 2008 22(6):621–632.

Grof, S. 'Varieties of Transpersonal experiences: Observations from LSD psychotherapy'. *Journal of Transpersonal Psychology.* 1972 4(2):45–80.

Grof, S. *Realms of the human unconscious: Observations from LSD research.* New York: Viking Press. 1975.

Grof, S. *LSD psychotherapy.* Pomona CA: Hunter House. 1980.

Grof, S. *The Adventure of Self Discovery.* Albany, NY: State University of New York Press. 1988.

Grof, S. *Psychology of the Future.* Albany, NY: State University of New York Press. 2000.

Grof, S. and Grof, C. *Holotropic Breathwork: a new approach to self-exploration and therapy.* New York: State University of New York Press. 2010.

Hood, R.W. 'The construction and preliminary validation of a measure of reported mystical experience'. *Journal for the Scientific Study of Religion.* 2006 14(1):29–41.

Hood, R.W. and Williamson, W.P. 'An empirical test of the unity thesis: The structure of mystical descriptors in various faith samples'. *Journal of Psychology and Christianity.* 2000 19(3):232–44.

James, W. *Las variedades de la experiencia religiosa*. Barcelona: Ed Peninsula. 1986.

Lukoff, D., Lu, F.G. 'Transpersonal psychology research review topic: mystical experience'. *Journal of Transpersonal Psychology*. 1988 20(2):161–184.

Pahnke, W.N. *Drugs and mysticism: an analysis of the relationship between psychedelic drugs and the mystical consciousness*. Unpublished doctoral thesis. Boston: Harvard University. 1963.

Pahnke, W.N. 'Drugs and Mysticism'. *International Journal of Parapsychology*. 1966 7(2):295–313.

Pahnke W.N. 'Psychedelic drugs and mystical experience'. *International Journal of Psychiatry in Clinical Practice*. 1969. (5):149–162.

Pahnke, W.N., Richards, W.A. 'Implications of LSD and experimental mysticism'. *Journal of Religion and Health*. 1966 5(3):175–208.

Puente, I. 'Holotropic breathwork can occasion mystical experiences in the context of a daylong workshop'. *Journal of Transpersonal Research*. 2015 6(2):40–50.

Richards, W.A. *Counselling, peak experiences and the human encounter with death: An empirical study of the efficacy of DPT assisted counselling in enhancing the quality of life of persons with terminal cancer and their closest family members*. PhD thesis. Washington DC: Catholic University of America. 1975.

Richards, W.A., Grof, S., Goodman, L., Kurland, A.A. 'LSD-assisted psychotherapy and the human encounter with death'. *Journal of Transpersonal Psychology*. 1972 4(2):121–150.

Richards, W.A., Rhead, J.C., Di Leo, F.B., Yensen, R., Kurland, A.A. 'The peak experience variable in DPT-assisted psychotherapy with cancer patients'. *Journal of Psychedelic Drugs*. 1977 9(1):1–10.

Stace, W.T. *Mysticism and Philosophy*. London: Ed McMillan. 1960.

Underhill, E. *Mysticism: the nature and development of spiritual*. 1993.

Zaehner, R.C. *Mysticism, Sacred and Profane: an inquiry into some varieties of praeternatural experience*. London: Oxford University Press. 1961.

PSYCHEDELICS AND NUMINOUS EXPERIENCE

TIM READ

Psychedelics bring the gift of numinous experience; there is simply no other method that provides such open access to high archetypal penetrance states. Numinous experiences are inherently challenging simply because they are so powerful. The term *numinous* implies an extra-ordinary mental state; a sense of awe, of enormity, of otherness. There is enormous potential for growth but the more powerful the instrument, the greater the risk of damage if the experience is insufficiently supported or integrated.

The quality of the experience depends on a number of factors, especially the drug itself, but there are some classical archetypal structures that may provide shape to the psychedelic experience. I will illustrate this with reference to the Promethean figures of Albert Hofmann, the chemist who first synthesised LSD and had the first intentional LSD experience, as well as the psychiatrist Stanislav Grof, who did extensive clinical research with LSD psychotherapy in the 1950s and 1960s.

AFTER THE BICYCLE RIDE

Being a scientific and methodical man, Albert Hofmann recorded taking 0.25 mg of lysergic acid diethylamide tartrate at 16.20. At 17.00

he reported dizziness, anxiety, visual distortions, symptoms of paralysis and desire to laugh. Then home by bicycle. From 18.00 to 20.00 the most severe crisis...[1]

Hofmann was escorted home by his laboratory assistant, who knew that he had taken an experimental substance. He felt threatened on the journey with distorted vision and a sensation of paralysis but according to his assistant they were travelling very rapidly. He made it home safely, summoned the family doctor and asked for milk as a non-specific antidote for poisoning.

What followed was horrible for him. Everything became threatening, even the furniture. His next-door neighbour bought him some milk but he perceived her as a malevolent witch with a coloured mask. But even worse than these 'demonic transformations of the outer world' were the alterations he perceived in his inner being. He felt utterly defeated by the drug, as though a demon had invaded and taken possession of him. He felt helpless, as though he was going insane. His body seemed lifeless and he thought he was dying. He was struck by the tragedy of the situation. His wife and three children had gone on a day trip and he describes intense guilt at leaving his young family behind. And it was his own entire fault through experimenting with this drug that he himself had brought into the world.

This marked the low point. By the time the doctor arrived, his despondency was easing. The doctor reassured him that his vital signs were stable, steered him to his bed and stayed with him. Hofmann describes how the horror softened, he felt the danger of insanity was past and he could allow himself to enjoy the experience, especially the kaleidoscopic visual imagery and the way sounds became transformed into colourful optical perceptions. His wife had been phoned to be told that he was having a breakdown, but by the time she arrived he was able to tell her what had happened. He slept soundly and awoke to find that the world was transformed.

A sensation of well-being and renewed life flowed through me. Breakfast tasted delicious and gave me extraordinary pleasure.

When I later walked out into the garden, in which the sun shone after a spring rain, everything glistened and sparkled in a fresh light. The world was as if newly created. All my senses vibrated in a condition of highest sensitivity, which persisted for the entire day.[2]

PSYCHEDELIC—ARCHAIDELIC

Psychedelics make us see things in a different way; they radically alter perspective and amplify our perception of meaning. The term psychedelic, means 'mind manifesting' but I have suggested that the term *archaidelic* may be more appropriate if these drugs create their effect by manifesting a specifically archetypal layer of psyche—a *high archetypal penetrance state.*[3]

Archetype is a mysterious concept. Archetypes are the great weather systems of meaning that are thought to represent deeper universal structures organised around significance and salience. Heightened exposure to the archetypal layer of consciousness holds a numinous quality—a sense of the sacred, whether deeply positive or terrifying—and this is one of the prime characteristics of the psychedelic experience. Numinous experience in various forms has always been prized by humanity although the Establishment is profoundly suspicious of it. You could say that numinous experience has been a crucial factor in the shaping of our collective human experience and culture.

Attempts to define archetypes present us with some difficulties if they are inherently unknowable and impossible to adequately describe. Historically we tried to understand them by personalising them as our Gods and Goddesses. Our understanding is deepened by the following five concepts:

- Plato's parable of the cave shows how we, the cave dwellers, are transfixed by the flickering shadows, the pale watered down version of the fundamental reality that lies beyond our everyday experience. The goal of the philosopher is to gain experience of the primary (archetypal) reality outside the cave. Ultimately everything emerges from the Sun, which represents the Self archetype.

- The theologian Rudolph Otto gives us the crucial notion of numinous experience as an *overplus of meaning*. The numinous is bivalent, having both light and dark manifestations, blissful or dreadful.
- Carl Jung learned from *synchronicity*, where there is a correspondence of meaning between the internal and external world, that archetypes are truly transpersonal constructs.
- The physicist David Bohm developed the *soma significance* model where meaning is an integral part of the physical universe. We could think of meaning as a fifth dimension that can be concentrated to an intensity that is beyond our capacity.
- Aldous Huxley popularised the concept of the brain as a *reducing valve*, so that our experience of meaning remains digestible and we are not overwhelmed.

There are a number of ways in which this hypothetical reducing valve can be bypassed to bring a greater intensity of meaning into our consciousness. We know that this occurs in various abnormal mental states that we classify as psychiatric illness. We also know that there are various techniques developed over millennia that have been prized for the ability to induce heightened meaning. These techniques include ritual, the use of sound, movement, meditation, fasting, prayer and psychoactive substances. Sometimes, these intense meaning states may come upon us spontaneously.

ENCOUNTER WITH SHADOW

The shadow is our dark side. It is the unseen reflection of the *persona*, which is the mask we use to present ourselves to the world. We all have a shadow; it is an inevitable part of being human. The shadow is the part of our psyche that is around the corner and hidden from our sight; it represents the part of ourselves that we do not choose to show to ourselves or anyone else. Milder forms of the encounter with the shadow may involve some low-mood, guilt, aggression or acting out but an encounter of archetypal intensity, as may occur with psychedelics, has a different quality altogether. Numinous shadow has an extraordinary quality of dreadfulness, hopelessness and evil.

The shadow is always by our side, requiring active suppression to keep it from our sight, and this acts as a drain on our psychological and energetic resources. If we can shine the light of conscious awareness into those dark places, if the shadow can be integrated and incorporated into a larger and more nuanced version of ourselves, we are immeasurably richer. Energy that was drained by defence mechanisms to protect the ego from the shadow can then be diverted to more creative use.

So we can gain hugely from processing shadow, but the encounter with the shadow is arguably the most challenging aspect of the psychedelic experience. It is not pleasant and in recreational use we would probably want to avoid it; but in therapeutic use and in a controlled setting it represents a wonderful opportunity to work with difficult and powerful unconscious psychic material that needs to be rendered conscious and integrated. This is the basis of psycholytic psychotherapy.[4]

Shadow is often projected onto the external environment. So in Hofmann's case, as the LSD began to bite and his ego defences dissolved, the surroundings became highly charged and threatening. His kindly neighbour who brought him his milk became suffused with demonic qualities that were a projection of Hofmann's own shadow. In other words, he did not realise that he was engaging with material from his own psyche and attributed his inner process (projected) to the external world. Then as he settled a little and became more tuned to his internal psychic processes he became preoccupied with his own sense of guilt, of abandoning and letting down his family and of failing in his professional life. He felt defeated and despairing.

The set and setting is of crucial importance in such situations. A mindset of tolerance, curiosity and enquiry combined with a supportive setting will generally allow the process to unfold so that the experience is negotiated safely and we emerge from darkness to sunlight. Indeed, this was Hofmann's experience. The article of faith in such archetypal crises is that the process, if adequately supported, is entirely natural, integrative and orientated towards our growth. The family doctor instinctively did exactly the right thing, he provided some reassurance that Hofmann did not seem in any physical danger and simply stayed with him. He was the world's first LSD sitter.

GROF AND THE PERINATAL ARCHETYPE

Stanislav Grof went to medical school with the intention of training as a psychoanalyst, but had a life-changing experience with his first LSD session in 1956 as part of a research project. His interest in psychiatry—which had been at an all-time low before this experience—got an enormous boost and he decided to dedicate his life to the study of non-ordinary states of consciousness.[5]

Grof describes a subsequent high dose LSD session where within an hour he was in a claustrophobic nightmare—a hellish no-exit situation with the ultimate existential crisis. He felt his entire existence was absurd and pointless. As well as feeling existentially trapped, he experienced a sense of pressure on his head and jaws. He felt crushed and had difficulties breathing. It suddenly came to him that he was reliving his biological birth. This very difficult LSD experience continued for about 3½ hours of clock time before suddenly opening up into light and bliss with a feeling that life was great and meaningful.

The original insight that Grof drew from this experience was that there was an aspect of his biological birth that had not been properly processed and was blocking his forward progress. He felt that on some level he was still trying to get out of the birth canal, and that this gestalt led to his feeling of always being on a treadmill and not be able to appreciate the present. Over subsequent years, working clinically with LSD psychotherapy with people with various states of emotional distress, Grof found that when people were able to relive and integrate their birth experience their symptoms seemed to resolve.[6]

Psychoanalytic theory at the time had been revolutionised by Melanie Klein's work on children. Klein's work showed how the emotional development of the newborn infant provided a template for psychological patterns that persisted into adult life.[7] But the assumption was that there were no significant psychological processes before birth; indeed Otto Rank had been excluded from Freud's inner circle for suggesting otherwise. But Grof has since developed his theories and arrived at some important conclusions:

- The birth process leaves its residue in adult psychological structures.
- The birth process can be accessed in states of non-ordinary consciousness.
- Working through perinatal issues can provide relief from a number of psychological and somatic ailments.
- These experiences have an archetypal quality.
- A re-enactment of the birth process in non-ordinary consciousness can act as a portal to transpersonal experience.

Taking the birth process from the perspective of the baby rather than that of the mother, four phases can be identified. To begin with there is the serenity of the womb, but this leads to the cataclysmic shock of the onset of labour, the struggle through the birth canal and the exhausted relief of delivery. These four distinctive meaning states comprise Grof's perinatal matrices.

The first perinatal matrix is the resting state that lasts until the onset of the contractions of labour. The baby develops peacefully in the amniotic sac with her entire needs being met by the encompassing and nourishing mother. Occasionally this resting state becomes poisonous, perhaps due to medication, toxins or lack of oxygen.

The second perinatal matrix is the physical onset of labour where the uterus contracts against a closed cervix. There is no available exit so this state involves an experience of constriction, entrapment and fear; the baby faces death.

The third perinatal matrix represents the physical process of movement out of constricted uterus through the opening cervix followed by the 'life or death struggle' through the birth canal. There is, after all, some light at the end of tunnel.

The fourth perinatal matrix is the birth, the emergence into the light, the first intake of breath and the recovery phase for mother and baby. The ordeal is over and they can meet each other for the first time in the outside world.

In the archetypal states that correspond to the perinatal journey, the first perinatal matrix involving good-womb experiences would equate to oceanic feelings of bliss and cosmic unity. A toxic womb state would equate to feeling in a bad place; poisoned or paranoid. The second perinatal matrix would involve profound hopelessness, despair and the encounter with death. This is the territory of the bad trip after the paradise of the first matrix is lost. The third perinatal matrix is the archetypal hero's journey, the call to arms, the tumultuous and perilous struggle. The fourth perinatal matrix holds themes of triumph, fortuitous escape from danger, revolution, decompression and expansion of space, radiant light and colour. This equates to Hofmann's radiant morning after the night before.

Grof found that the perinatal matrices and their archetypal manifestations are most vividly encountered in states of non-ordinary consciousness, but that they also occur in routine clinical situations and are insufficiently understood by contemporary psychiatry. In charting this archetypal perinatal journey, Grof provides a route map to guide us through these challenging 'bad trip' experiences so that we may gradually process these layers of trauma and emerge reborn. Sometimes this can occur in the space of one session, as with Hofmann; but often it takes longer.

THE ARCHETYPE OF EGO DEATH AND REBIRTH

We are brought up to identify with the ego structures that we have to develop to navigate our way in the world. We become very attached to these structures, particularly as they solidify after adolescence. Psychedelics have an ego dissolving effect, which is dose related.

No other class of drugs has quite the same effect on ego structures. With high dose LSD the psychic apparatus that we depend on for everyday use simply does not function for us any more. Sometimes, particularly for inexperienced psychedelic explorers or for people with rigid ego defences, this is associated with a feeling that real and physical death is imminent. This was certainly the case for Hofmann, who was convinced that he was dying. This can be dangerous and as a psychiatrist working in a trauma unit, I have seen a number of people in states of archetypal crisis who have confused ego death with physical death and tried to take their own lives. In Grof's terminology these psychological states correspond to the second matrix and are particularly difficult to treat due to the sheer perception of hopelessness and prevailing mood of cynicism and meaninglessness. There is an archetypal amplification of catastrophe; it feels as though titanic forces are ranged against you. There really is no exit and no point in trying to find one.

But usually the crisis passes and something extraordinary seems to happen. The dis-identification with our egoic structures and layers of conditioning allows an opening to something that is invigorating and generally has a profound spiritual charge. This mysterious source of energy and inspiration has many names but from an archetypal psychology perspective it is termed the Self. The Self is at the apex of the pyramid of archetypes; indeed, it is beyond archetype, for it is the primal unity from which archetypes flow. The Self is comparable to the Hindu concept of Atman. For the Hindus, Atman pervades us utterly, as Krishna tells the hero of the Bhagavad Gita: 'I am the Self in the heart of every creature, Arjuna, and the beginning, middle and end of their existence'.[8] From this perspective, the Self never leaves us, but is merely repressed by development of the ego structures.

The religious scholar John Huston Smith gives a vivid account of an encounter with Self during his first LSD experience provided by Timothy Leary. Having spent 10 years trying and failing to find cosmic consciousness through Zen Buddhism, he found with LSD that he ascended step-by-step 'to those things on which angels themselves long to gaze'.[9] He had the thought that if he took the last step and merged with the all-consuming limitless bliss, that he would die. And he warned Leary that he could have a corpse on his hands. Presumably Leary was used to this sort of psychedelic death pronouncement.

Huston Smith had no doubt that his experience of cosmic consciousness was entirely valid, an authentic religious experience. The day after his first LSD session he wrote that overnight he had become a visionary, he not only believed in the larger world but had actually visited it.[10] Smith discontinued psychedelics after about half a dozen sessions, finding that the usefulness seemed to go down and the bummers increased. As someone who was more interested in cosmic insights than his own personal unconscious, he didn't find the challenging 'negative' experiences of much interest. But I wonder if he could have profited more from the opportunities to process shadow that these bummers were offering him.

MIND THE STEP, OPEN THE DOORS

In dissolving ego structures, we can open to the primal energies of Self. As the process evolves, the ego emerges again, but in reconstituted form. It is an ego suffused with Self and the world is wonderfully transformed. This is a complicated process and for many of us it may take some time and repeated experiences. It may have the flavour of two steps forward and one step back, for the ego is resilient and does not easily give ground. This is the stuff of the classic midlife crisis; a crisis of meaning where the ego structures that have served their purpose well over the first part of life become less useful and need to be re-arranged. Sometimes this process flows smoothly, but the ego tends to resist this process strongly. The midlife crisis (which can occur at any age from adolescence onwards) then develops as a battle between the ego that was and the reconstituted ego that needs to be brought into being. It is a battle of ego death and rebirth. I suggest that non-ordinary states of consciousness are of great value in negotiating the midlife crisis; the key to the process is supporting the failure of ego structures while facilitating an opening to Self.[11]

This engagement with the Self archetype is of huge significance both on a personal and a collective level. We may find ourselves moving decisively away from our cultural conditioning and taking new perspectives suffused with Self energy. Typically, we disown the more masculine, martial, thrusting qualities and become more open to qualities of love, harmony and co-operation. Indeed the term *femtheogen* has been coined to describe the way that psychedelics allow access to the numinous feminine principle (anima) to act as a bridge between ego and Self.[12] Perhaps the most obvious example of this was the anti-war movement in the 1960s, fuelled by the expansion of consciousness associated with LSD, which so profoundly challenged the political establishment. This led to the criminalisation of LSD, which lost us the potential therapeutic effects of these drugs for a couple of generations.

Positively charged high archetypal penetrance states also amplify our perception of beauty. Huxley coined the term positive transfiguration to describe how light spills out of the interior world into the external world so that it seems overwhelmingly beautiful, alive and shining.[13] This tends to lead to an enhanced appreciation of nature and our relationship with it. Hofmann felt that many people were blocked, without an inborn facility to realise beauty, and it is these people who may need a psychedelic experience to have a visionary experience of nature.[14]

It is not necessary to have the classic death/rebirth sequence in order to access the spiritual and transformative energies of the Self. But many of us need to go through this shadow processing experience, at least to some extent, in order to bypass the blocks presented by our conditioning, our traumas and our appetites. It is a wonderful gift to have the beautiful moments, to touch the stars, to play with the angels— but in order to see and hear in different ways, we may also need to do some work on the ways in which we may be blind or deaf, figuratively speaking. It is because we are sometimes so defended that we actually need these more challenging experiences to open our eyes, to cleanse the doors of perception. But in order to make use of them we really do need an enquiring and open mindset, a highly supportive setting and the tools to process and integrate the material into consciousness so that it is of use. If we are going to have a numinous experience of the darker variety, we would do well to embrace it. And we need to be prepared to do some work on it; experience without integration is an opportunity wasted.

References:

1. Hofmann, A. *LSD: My Problem Child*. Sarasota, FL: MAPS. 1979.

2. Ibid. 50.

3. Read, T. *Walking Shadows*. London: Muswell Hill Press. 2014.

4. Meckel Fischer, F. *Therapy with Substance*. Muswell Hill Press: London. 2015.

5. Grof, S. In *Higher wisdom: Eminent Elders Explore the Continuing Impact of Psychedelics*. Walsh, R., Grob, C. (eds). New York: SUNY. 2005. 51.

6. Grof, S. *Realms of the Human Unconscious: Observations from LSD Research*. New York: Viking. 1975.

7. Klein, M. 'Our Adult World and its Roots in Infancy'. *Human Relations*. November 1959. Vol. 12 no. 4, 291–303.

8. Easwaran, E. *The Bhagavad Gita*. Nilgiri. 1985. 2.

9. Smith, H. *In Higher wisdom: Eminent Elders Explore the Continuing Impact of Psychedelics*. Walsh, R., Grob, C. (eds). New York: SUNY. 2005. 225.

10. Smith, H. *Tales of Wonder*. New York: HarperCollins. 2009.

11. Read, T. 'Archetypal Penetrance and the Midlife Crisis'. *Network Review*. Spring 2016. 3.

12. Papaspyrou, M. 'Femtheogens'. In *Out of the Shadows*. Dickens, R., Read, T. (eds). London: Muswell Hill Press. 2015.

13. Huxley, A. *Moksha*. Rochester, Vermont: Park Street Press. 1977. 204.

14. Hofmann, A. In *Higher wisdom: Eminent Elders Explore the Continuing Impact of Psychedelics*. Walsh, R., Grob, C. (eds). New York: SUNY. 2005. 51.

ACKNOWLEDGEMENTS

Enormous praise goes to my fellow Breaking Convention Executive Committee members, Cameron Adams, David King, David Luke and Aimee Tollan—the book's co-editors—for their shared responsibility of peer-reviewing this volume of essays, and Nikki Wyrd for proofreading the selections.

Ongoing thanks, as ever, to the wider Breaking Convention crew of Mark Lewis, Maria Papaspyrou, Stephen Reid, Julian Vayne, Andy Roberts, Ashleigh Murphy, Alexander Beiner, Cara Lavan, Adam Malone, Hattie Wells, Hayley Cattlin, Robert Dickins, Stuart Griggs —for keeping the wheels turning and the conferences alive.

Thanks to Mark Pilkington and Tihana Šare at Strange Attractor Press for sticking with us for this third volume. I am glad you agreed with the groovy Clear Light white cover.

An exceptional mention to Rob Dickins and the crew at Psychedelic Press for bringing out a special edition of your journal to include those authors whose valuable works we could not fit into this book.

And finally, tremendous thanks to all the contributors of those vital words who actually wrote the book.

See you all in at BC17—and beyond!

Ben Sessa

EDITORIAL TEAM

Lead Editor: Ben Sessa

With Co-Editors: David Luke, Aimee Tollan, David King, Cameron Adams and Nikki Wyrd.

Lead Editor

Ben Sessa is a consultant child and adolescent psychiatrist working in adult addictions and with young offenders. Ben is interested in the developmental trajectory from child maltreatment to adult mental disorders and addictions. Since 2009 Ben has administered and received legal doses of LSD, psilocybin, MDMA, DMT and Ketamine as senior research fellow at Bristol and Imperial College London Universities and is currently conducting the UK's first two clinical studies with MDMA-assisted therapy for the treatment of PTSD and alcohol use disorder. Ben has authored peer-reviewed articles in the mainstream medical press and written several books, including *The Psychedelic Renaissance* (2012 & 2017), *Psychedelic Drug Treatments* (with Eileen Worthey, 2016) and *To Fathom Hell or Soar Angelic* (2015). Alongside his supervisor, David Nutt, Ben lobbies for a change to drug prohibition policies that increase the harms of drug use and stifle opportunities for psychedelic research. He is a co-founder and current president of Breaking Convention. www.drsessa.com

Co-Editors

David Luke, PhD, is Senior Lecturer in Psychology at the University of Greenwich, where he hosts Breaking Convention, the organisation that he cofounded and is a director of. His research focuses on transpersonal experiences, anomalous phenomena and altered states of consciousness, especially via psychedelics, having published more than 100 academic papers in this area, including seven books, most recently *Otherworlds: Psychedelics and Exceptional Human Experience* (Muswell Hill, 2017). He also founded and directs the Ecology, Cosmos and Consciousness salon in London.

Aimée Tollan is an Anthropology graduate from the University of Kent, the home of the first Breaking Convention. She joined the UKC Psychedelics Society which is where she became initiated into the psychedelic community. She has been involved in Breaking Convention from the start, firstly as a volunteer and then was invited on to the Executive Committee in late 2013. Her main area of interest is drug policy reform which inspired her undergraduate dissertation exploring public attitudes towards drugs. Residing in London, her current thoughts are concerned with the lack of diversity within the psychedelic community.

Dave King is a graduate medical student at King's College London and holds a BSc in Medical Anthropology. He is a founding co-director of Breaking Convention and a co-director of the Scientific & Medical Network. As founding President of the King's College Society for Psychedelic Studies, Dave co-hosts a Drug-Assisted Psychotherapies Programme at the Institute of Psychiatry, Psychology & Neuroscience. He also co-founded the UK's first academic student psychedelics society at the University of Kent in 2008, and now chairs a consortium of UK-based student psychedelic groups. He has published a number of scientific, literary and opinion articles and is a co-editor of the three Breaking Convention anthologies.

Cameron Adams is a founding co-director of Breaking Convention. He is a medical and cognitive anthropologist with interests in self-healing, the politics of health, biopower, social aspects of health and wellbeing with special reference to psychedelics as well as social exclusion and its role in negative psychedelic experiences such as paranoia, anxiety and conspiracy mentation. In addition to co-editing the three Breaking Convention anthologies, he has published several articles, including: 'Psychedelics and Shadows of Society' (*openDemocracy*), 'Cultural Variation in the Apparent Jungian Archetype of the Feminine in Psychedelic Personification' (*Proceedings of Daimonic Imagination: Uncanny Intelligence*), 'From Meta-Sin to Medicine: A Program for Future Research Psychedelics as Medicine' (*Proceedings of the Breaking Convention: Multidisciplinary Conference on Psychedelic Consciousness*), 'Medicine, Healing and Psychedelics' (*The Meanings of High: Variations According to Drug, Time, Set and Setting*), 'Psychedelics, Spirits and the Sacred Feminine: Communion as Cultural Critique' (*Paranthropology: Journal of Anthropological Approaches to the Paranormal*).

Nikki Wyrd (BSc, Ecology) is a freelance proofreader and copy editor. She works with a wide range of clients, specializing in health, science and psychedelic related topics, and is the current Editor of the *Psychedelic Press Journal*. She also publishes thought-provoking books, gives lectures, and facilitates workshops and retreats focusing on self-realization. She is also known for her capability as a ritualist and an event host in occult circles. Having shown herself to be an invaluable asset in the smooth functioning of Breaking Convention, she was invited onto the Directors' committee in 2015. Nikki's quest is to improve the world, by helping others to share practices which allow each of us to improve our lives. Her best work as a writer is yet to come.

CONTRIBUTORS

Sam Gandy has had a lifelong interest in nature and wildlife and in more recent years this fascination has extended to consciousness and altered states. His academic background is in physical geography, ecology and entomology and he is currently in the latter stages of a PhD in Ecological Science at The University of Aberdeen. He has a love of travelling the world, and through research has been very fortunate in having the opportunity to work in Peru, Kefalonia, Spain, Vietnam, Texas and Brazil. His current research is focussed on soils, termites, ecosystem services and soil rehabilitation in southern Ethiopia, where he has spent half a year. Research and nature aside, he has a passion for writing and science communication and has contributed to a number of publications and spoken at a number of conferences, festivals and fairs.

Allan Badiner is a contributing editor at *Tricycle* magazine, and the editor of the new edition of *Zig Zag Zen: Buddhism and Psychedelics* (Synergetic Press). He also edited the books, *Dharma Gaia: A Harvest in Buddhism and Ecology*, and *Mindfulness in the Marketplace* (Parallax Press). His written work appears in other books including *Dharma Family Treasures, Meeting the Buddha, Ecological Responsibility: A Dialogue with Buddhism*, and *The Buddha and the Terrorist*. Allan holds a Masters from the College of Buddhist Studies in LA and serves on the boards of Rainforest Action Network, and Project CBD.

Friederike Meckel Fischer, MD, trained as a medical doctor and a medical psychotherapist in Germany. She trained as a Holotropic Breathwork© facilitator with Prof. Stanislav Grof in the US. Friederike realised the additional therapeutic benefits of psychoactive substances through her own experiences. She was lucky to join a psychotherapeutic training group in substance supported psychotherapy. She is also trained in couples councelling, family therapy and family-constellation. She worked in her own private (psychotherapeutic) practice for almost 20 years. Over a couple of years she developed her specific way of substance supported psychotherapy, working underground with specially chosen clients in groups. Today she no longer does substance supported psychotherapy. Being retired she still offers some private counselling in Zürich. Her book *Therapy with Substance* was published in 2015. She is an advocate of substance supported therapy, a reminder of the indivisible unity of body, mind and soul on the way to the authentic personality in everyday spirituality.

Tharcila Chaves is a pharmacist with a master's degree in medicine and sociology of drug abuse. Currently, she is a PhD student at the University of Groningen (North Netherlands) and also an editor of the OPEN Foundation (psychedelic research association of the Netherlands). In her master's degree, she conducted a qualitative study about cravings in crack cocaine users in the city of São Paulo (Brazil). The use of ketamine to treat pain and depression is the focus of her current research.

John Constable is a playwright, poet and performer. His many plays include *Black Mass, Tulip Futures*, and *The Southwark Mysteries*, received in a vision on 23rd November 1996 and performed in Shakespeare's Globe and Southwark Cathedral. Solo work includes *I Was An Alien Sex God* and *Spare*, inspired by the life and work of Austin Osman

Spare. He is also widely known as John Crow, the urban shaman who raised the spirit of The Goose at Cross Bones, south London's outcasts' graveyard. In this magical persona, he conducts *The Halloween of Cross Bones* and vigils at Cross Bones, where he has created a shrine and a garden of remembrance. His Sha-Manic Plays, *The Southwark Mysteries* and his stage adaptation of Mervyn Peake's *Gormenghast* are all published by Oberon Books. A collection of his poetry, *Spark In The Dark*, is published by Thin Man Books. For more information: www. crossbones.org.uk

Lorna Olivia O'Dowd, PhD, is a psychotherapist.

Rick Doblin, PhD, is the founder and executive director of the Multidisciplinary Association for Psychedelic Studies (MAPS). He received his doctorate in Public Policy from Harvard's Kennedy School of Government, where he wrote his dissertation on the regulation of the medical uses of psychedelics. His undergraduate thesis at New College of Florida was a 25-year follow-up to the classic Good Friday Experiment, which evaluated the potential of psychedelic drugs to catalyse religious experiences. Rick studied with Dr Stanislav Grof and was among the first to be certified as a Holotropic Breathwork practitioner. His professional goal is to help develop legal contexts for the beneficial uses of psychedelics and marijuana, primarily as prescription medicines but also for personal growth for otherwise healthy people, and eventually to become a legally licensed psychedelic therapist. He founded MAPS in 1986, and currently resides in Boston with his wife and one of three children (two in college).

Amanda Feilding is the Founder and Director of the Beckley Foundation. Amanda established the foundation in 1998 to further research into the therapeutic and transformative potential of psychoactive substances forbidden by prohibitionist policies, and has since been called the 'hidden hand behind the renaissance of psychedelic science and drug policy reform.' Through the Scientific

Programme, Amanda directs collaborations with leading scientists worldwide, investigating cannabis, psilocybin, LSD, Ayahuasca, DMT and MDMA. These include clinical trials identifying the effects of psychoactive substances on cerebral circulation, brain function, subjective experience, and clinical symptoms. She co-directs the thriving Beckley/Imperial Research Programme with Professor David Nutt.

Mike Crowley was born in Wales and, in the mid-1960s, encountered psychedelics and Buddhism. A chance meeting with a Tibetan lama in London led to his becoming a lay-member of the Kagyud order in 1970. Following intense practice and study, Mike was ordained as a lama in 1987. Mike has lectured on Buddhist epistemology at the Jagellonian University, Cracow, Poland, on Tibetan history at the Museum of Asia and the Pacific, Warsaw, Poland and on various aspects of Buddhist practice at the Polish National Buddhist Center. He has also presented at various conferences including Mind States (San Francisco), Entheogenesis (Vancouver, BC), Sacred Elixirs (San Jose, California) and Breaking Convention (Canterbury, UK). He now lives in rural seclusion in the Shasta-Trinity National Forest, northern California.

Robert Dickins is a historian, writer and editor. He is the founder of the Psychedelic Press, co-director of the Psychedelic Museum, and is currently undertaking his PhD at Queen Mary, University of London. His research interests focus on the history and literature of psychedelic substances, and the role of writing in spiritual and magical traditions during the 19th century. He is also the author of the novel *Erin*, and has occasionally been known to perform a poem or two.

Luke Goaman-Dodson is a writer and researcher based in the South East of England. He holds an MA in Comparative Literature from the University of Kent.

Ido Hartogsohn, PhD, is a historian and sociologist of psychedelics and culture. His thesis *The Psycho-Social Construction of LSD: How Set and Setting Shaped the American Psychedelic Experience 1950–1970* explored the role of society and culture in shaping the results of mid-twentieth century American psychedelic research and the reception of psychedelics into American culture. Over the years Hartogsohn has written and published extensively on the topic of psychedelics in Israeli and international media. Among other things, he is the editor of the Israeli psychedelic magazine *La Psychonaut* and the founder and chief-editor of psychedelic video collection dailypsychedelicvideo.com. Hartogsohn's book *Technomysticism: Technology and Consciousness in the Digital Age* (Madaf, 2009: Hebrew) received much acclaim and was among the first works to introduce the subject of psychedelia to the Israeli public. He is currently completing his book project *American Trip: How Set and Setting Shaped the American Psychedelic Experience.*

Scott J. Hill, PhD, conducts independent scholarly research on the intersection between Jungian psychology and psychedelic studies. He holds degrees in psychology and educational psychology from the University of Minnesota, and a PhD from the California Institute of Integral Studies in San Francisco. He is the author of *Confrontation with the Unconscious: Jungian Depth Psychology and Psychedelic Experience.*

William Rowlandson is Senior Lecturer in Hispanic Studies at the University of Kent. He is the author of *Imaginal Landscapes* (Swedenborg Society, 2015), *Borges, Swedenborg and Mysticism* (Peter Lang, 2013), *Reading Lezama's 'Paradiso'* (Peter Lang, 2007), and co-editor with Angela Voss of *Daimonic Imagination: Uncanny Intelligence* (Cambridge Scholars, 2013). He has published widely on Latin American cultural and political history, and has published various translations from Spanish into English. He is a regular contributor to *Paranthropology: Journal of Anthropological Approaches to the Paranormal.* He plays drums as often as he can. www. williamrowlandson.wordpress.com

David E. Nichols, PhD, is currently an Adjunct Professor in the Eshelman School of Pharmacy at the University of North Carolina, Chapel Hill, NC. The focus of his graduate training, beginning in 1969, and of most of his research subsequent to receiving his doctorate in 1973 has been the investigation of the relationship between molecular structure and the action of various substances that modify behavioural states. A major focus of his research was on substances known as hallucinogens, or more popularly as psychedelics. His research was continuously funded by government agencies for three decades. Widely published in the scientific literature and internationally recognised for his research on centrally active drugs, he has studied all of the major classes of psychedelic agents, including LSD and other lysergic acid derivatives, psilocybin and the tryptamines, and phenethylamines related to mescaline. Among scientists, he is recognized as one of the foremost experts on the medicinal chemistry of hallucinogens.

Jennifer Lyke is a counselling psychologist and Associate Professor of Psychology at Richard Stockton University in New Jersey. She teaches courses in consciousness and anomalous experiences to undergraduates and sees clients in private practice. Her research interests include altered states of consciousness, especially mystical experiences, and factors related to psychopathology. She has published articles on topics such as peak experiences induced by psilocybin, mediumship and mysticism, and personality characteristics related to clinical symptoms. She resides in the United States.

Julia Kuti was an undergraduate psychology major at Stockton University at the time of this research. She has since graduated and pursued various professional opportunities in France, Utah, and South America. She remains interested in neuroscience and studying psychedelics.

Michael Montagne, PhD, is a drug researcher working in Boston, Mass. Educated in pharmacy and sociology he then received postdoctoral training in psychiatric epidemiology at Johns Hopkins

University. He is the author of over 300 research publications, over 40 book chapters, and four books including: *Searching for Magic Bullets: Orphan Drugs, Consumer Activism, and Pharmaceutical Development,* 1994. He has written for the *Psychozoic Press, Psychedelic Monographs & Essays, Integration,* and the *Psychedelic Press UK.* He has taught and performed research for 40 years on the social, cultural, and historical aspects of the drug experience. He can be reached at: mecm6634@gmail.com.

Jonathan Newman is an anthropological investigator interested in the contested moral and economic values of commodities. His explorations, so far, have taken him into three economic sectors—coffee, drugs and security. Subsequently, he has published elements of his research within each industry—*The Longberry, Weed World,* and *City Security Magazine.* Other publications include the *New Statesman, Emergency Medicine Journal* and *Third World Quarterly.* The research interest in drugs derived from talking to cannabis breeders and other cannabis professionals who support the Medical Cannabis Bike Tour. Jonathan is writing a book about his drugs research and also producing a collection of articles on a diversity of anthropological encounters from gravity to tidying. In 2018, he returns to the field again, together with Noodles the dog. They will attempt to discover a route for anthropology to bypass institutional power and arrive at everyday practice.

Carl A.P. Ruck is Professor of Classics at Boston University, an authority on the ecstatic rituals of the god Dionysus. With the ethno-mycologist R. Gordon Wasson and Albert Hofmann, he identified the secret psychoactive ingredient in the visionary potion that was drunk by the initiates at the Eleusinian Mystery. In *Persephone's Quest: Entheogens and the Origins of Religion,* he proclaimed the centrality of psychoactive sacraments at the very beginnings of religion, employing the neologism 'entheogen' to free the topic from the pejorative connotations for words like drug or hallucinogen. His publications include: *Mushrooms, Myth, and Mithras: The Drug Cult that Civilized*

Europe; The Effluents of Deity: Alchemy and Psychoactive Sacraments in Medieval and Renaissance Art; Sacred Mushrooms of the Goddess: Secrets of Eleusis; Entheogens, Myth and Human Consciousness; Dionysus in Thrace; The Son Conceived in Drunkenness; The Great Gods of Samothrace and the Cult of the Little People.

Dale Pendell, poet and scientist, is the author of over a dozen books of poetry, fiction, and non-fiction. He hails from a woodsy hill on a Mesozoic reversely-zoned gabbro-diorite pluton in the Sierra Nevada of California. More at dalependell.com

Alan Piper has a special interest in the hidden history of psychedelic culture. Published papers include 'Leo Perutz and the Mystery of *St Peter's Snow*', which concerns an Austrian novel from 1933 that contains a mysteriously detailed prediction of the discovery of LSD and refers to a hidden history of ergot as a secret Gnostic sacrament, 'A 1920's Harvard Psychedelic Circle with a Mormon Connection' in the journal *Invisible College*, and 'The Mysterious Origins of the Word 'Marihuana''. Alan's review of Ernst Jünger's novel *Visit to Godenholm*, which was based in part on LSD sessions Jünger shared with Albert Hofmann, can be found on the Psypress website. 'The Altered States of David Lindsay: Three Psychedelic Novels of the 1920s' appeared in *Psychedelic Press* journal Volume XX. Published papers by Alan, together with the slides and video links, for his two Breaking Convention presentations, can be found online through academia.edu. Occasional unpublished papers can be found at https://tzanjo.wordpress.com

Graham St John, PhD, is an Australian cultural anthropologist specialising in event-cultural movements and entheogens. Among his eight books are *Mystery School in Hyperspace: A Cultural History of DMT* (North Atlantic Books 2015), *Global Tribe: Technology, Spirituality and Psytrance* (Equinox 2012), and *Technomad: Global Raving Countercultures* (Equinox 2009). He works in the Dept of

Social Science, University of Fribourg, Switzerland, as Senior Research Fellow on the SNSF project Burning Progeny: The European Efflorescence of Burning Man. He is Executive Editor of *Dancecult: Journal of Electronic Dance Music Culture*. His website is: www.edgecentral.net

Bruce Rimell is an independent researcher and visual artist whose work explores the interplay between the visionary, the evolutionary, the anthropological and the cognitive. He is currently developing a philosophy of 'Visionary Humanism', an attempt to bridge the gaps between science and spirituality, by surpassing contemporary antagonisms through explorations into human symbolic thought and the creation of new 'cognitive/evolutionary' visionary epistemologies. To this end, he has published two books, *On Vision and Being Human*, an initial statement on the philosophy, and *Liminal Contact*, in which the philosophy is applied to art and painting. A third book, *They Shimmer Within*, a cognitive model of visionary beings and other supernatural agents, is currently in progress. He is a Fellow of the Royal Society of the Arts in the UK, and a member of several international arts networks, and has presented his research to diverse range audiences including queer theory and psychedelic/visionary conferences worldwide and the Radical Anthropology Group in London.

Iker Puente is psychologist, researcher and writer. He obtained his PhD degree at the UAB with his dissertation 'Complexity and Transpersonal Psychology: chaos, self-organization and peak experiences in psychotherapy', exploring the short and medium term effects and the subjective effects of different breathwork techniques. He has been trained in Gestalt Therapy, Integrative Bodywork Therapy and in Holotropic Breathwork and Transpersonal Psychology. He has been visiting scholar at the California Institute of Integral Studies (CIIS), a member of the psychedelic emergency service at Boom Festival and other festivals since in 2008, and has teaching experience in the field of transpersonal psychology. He works as a psychotherapist in Barcelona, organise breathwork workshops and transpersonal psychology seminars and courses. He is also Assistant Editor of the Journal of Transpersonal Research (JTR), and a founding member of the Ibero-American Transpersonal Association (ATI). He recently published his first book *Psychedelic psychotherapy and research: past, present and future.*

Tim Read is a medical doctor, psychiatrist and psychotherapist based in London. He was Consultant Psychiatrist at the Royal London Hospital for 20 years. He has trained in psychoanalytic therapy (IGA) and in transpersonal therapy (GTT) with Stanislav Grof. He is a co-founder of the Institute of Transpersonal and Archetypal Studies (ITAS) and a certified facilitator of Holotropic Breathwork. Tim also co-founded Muswell Hill Press and his book *Walking Shadows: Archetype and Psyche in Crisis and Growth* was published in 2014.

STRANGE ATTRACTOR PRESS 2017